Angina Pectoris in Clinical Practice

Edited by

PETER M SCHOFIELD MD FRCP FICA FACC FESC
CONSULTANT CARDIOLOGIST
CARDIAC UNIT
PAPWORTH HOSPITAL
PAPWORTH EVERARD
CAMBRIDGE

MARTIN DUNITZ

© Martin Dunitz Ltd 1999

First published in the United Kingdom in 1999 by
Martin Dunitz Ltd
The Livery House
7–9 Pratt Street
London NW1 0AE

Tel: +44-(0)171-482-2202
Fax: +44-(0)171-267-0159
E-mail: info@mdunitz.globalnet.co.uk
Website: http://www.dunitz.co.uk

A CIP catalogue record for this book is available from the British Library

ISBN 1-85317-720-2

Distributed in the United States by:
Blackwell Science Inc.
Commerce Place, 350 Main Street
Malden MA 02148, USA
Tel: 1-800-215-1000

Distributed in Canada by:
Login Brothers Book Company
324 Salteaux Crescent
Winnipeg, Manitoba R3J 3T2
Canada
Tel: 1-204-224-4068

Distributed in Brazil by:
Ernesto Reichmann Distribuidora de Livros, Ltda
Rua Coronel Marques 335, Tatuape 03440–000
Sao Paulo
Brazil

Composition by Wearset, Boldon, Tyne and Wear
Printed and bound in Spain by Grafos, S.A. Arte Sobre papel

Contents

Contributors

Martin R Bennett PhD MRCP
British Heart Foundation Senior Fellow / Honorary
Consultant Cardiologist, Department of Medicine,
Addenbrooke's Hospital, Cambridge CB2 2QQ.

Paul D Flynn MB BChir MA MRCP(UK) MRCPI
Clinical Lecturer, Department of Medicine, University of
Cambridge, and Honorary Specialist Registrar,
Addenbrooke's Hospital, Cambridge CB2 2QQ.

Samer A M Nashef MB ChB FRCS
Consultant Cardiothoracic Surgeon, Papworth Hospital,
Papworth Everard, Cambridge CB3 8RE.

Edward Rowland MB BS MD FACC FESC
Consultant Cardiologist, Department of Cardiological
Sciences, St George's Hospital Medical School, London
SW17 0RE.

Peter M Schofield MD FRCP FICA FACC FESC
Consultant Cardiologist, Cardiac Unit, Papworth Hospital,
Papworth Everard, Cambridge CB3 8RE.

Leonard M Shapiro BSc MD FRCP FACC
Consultant Cardiologist, Cardiac Unit,
Papworth Hospital, Papworth Everard,
Cambridge CB3 8RE.

Paul W L Siklos MA BSc MBBS FRCP
Consultant Physician, West Suffolk Hospital,
Department of Adult Medicine, Bury St
Edmunds, Suffolk IP33 2QZ.

David L Stone BSc MD FRCP
Consultant Cardiologist, Cardiac Unit,
Papworth Hospital, Papworth Everard,
Cambridge CB3 8RE.

Peter L Weissberg MD FRCP FESC FMedSci
British Heart Foundation Professor of
Cardiovascular Medicine, University of
Cambridge School of Clinical Medicine,
Department of Medicine, Addenbrooke's
Hospital, Cambridge CB2 2QQ.

Yee Guan Yap BMedSci MB BS MRCP,
British Heart Foundation Research Fellow in
Cardiology, Department of Cardiological
Sciences, St George's Hospital Medical
School, London SW17 0RE.

Foreword

Angina pectoris (from the Latin for 'strangling in the chest') is rarely very painful as sufferers stop what they are doing before it becomes so. For many patients with stable angina it is simply a mild pressure which greets them like an old friend after walking a certain distance, but a common accompaniment of this symptom is fear. This is heightened when patients realize that the onset of angina marks that moment in their lives when their coronary arterial disease has started to compromise myocardial blood flow and hence their prognosis. Herein lies the importance of this book, which is devoted to the identification and management of patients with angina pectoris.

The epidemiology and natural history of angina pectoris are now well known although the diagnostic tools, drug treatment and techniques for myocardial revascularization are changing rapidly. Particular examples include the use of stress echocardiography in diagnosis, the impact of statins on prognosis, the value of potassium channel opening drugs for symptom relief, minimally invasive cardiac surgery and laser revascularization.

Angina Pectoris in Clinical Practice is a timely and welcome addition to the cardiological literature. It should sit on a nearby shelf in the general practitioner's office, in the physician's clinic, in the coronary care unit and wherever doctors, nurses, rehabilitation workers and others have responsibility for those suffering from angina. Thereby the prognosis and well-being of their patients can be improved.

Michael C Petch MD, FRCP, FACC, FESC
Consultant Cardiologist
Papworth Hospital
Cambridge

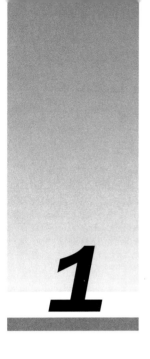

Clinical history and examination (including risk factors, epidemiology and aetiology)

Paul W L Siklos

Introduction

The aim of this chapter is to enable the reader to establish a diagnosis of angina pectoris from the patient's symptoms. In order to do this it is important to consider the geographical distribution of and risk factors for ischaemic heart disease (IHD) (the commonest cause of angina) because consideration of the frequency with which a condition appears in a population gives a strong indication as to the likelihood that a given symptom, sign or test result is significant in diagnosis. For example, 'typical anginal pain' in a 25-year-old girl is unlikely to be due to IHD, whereas the converse is true of a 55-year-old man who smokes cigarettes and complains of similar symptoms.

Aetiology

Angina pectoris is chest discomfort caused by myocardial ischaemia, so any situation which increases myocardial work and oxygen consumption, or reduces oxygenation or (usually) both, will cause angina. The commonest underlying cause is atheromatous epicardial coronary artery disease, which must narrow the coronary artery by at least 50–70% of its luminal diameter before reduction in coronary bloodflow is likely to cause symptoms.

However, it is important to remember the following which may cause (or contribute to) angina:

• aortic stenosis;
• pulmonary hypertension;
• hypertrophic cardiomyopathy;
• anaemia, polycythaemia;
• tachycardia — primary electrical abnormality or secondary to hyperthyroid state or fever;
• coronary arteritis;
• coronary artery spasm;
• variant (Prinzmetal) angina — spontaneous development of chest discomfort with ST elevation on the electrocardiogram;
• syndrome X — angina accompanied by evidence of myocardial ischaemia such as ST depression on the electrocardiogram but with 'normal' coronary arteries (there may be 'small vessel disease').

The association of 'typical angina' with coronary artery disease is stronger in men than in women, with up to half of women referred for coronary angiography having normal epicardial coronary arteries. There is also evidence that vasospasm and microvascular disease are more common in women and cause atypical pain.

Epidemiology

Cardiovascular disease is the major cause of death in adults (approximately 40% of all-cause mortality before the age of 74 years) in the majority of developed countries and in some that are developing, and most of this disease is attributable to atherosclerosis. Epidemiological studies aim to document the amount of this disease and its distribution for economic purposes and to help determine cause. All European countries submit annual mortality data to the World Health Organization and these data were recently published.[1] The age-standardized mortality for IHD for men aged 45–74 years varied between 907 deaths a year per 100 000 population in Latvia to 142 in France, with a similar east–west gradient for women of the same age (342 deaths per year per 100 000 in Ukraine and 36 in France). In addition, there is a north–south gradient in the UK and France with highest mortality in the north. The annual percentage change in mortality from IHD between 1970 and 1992 again shows that eastern Europe is disadvantaged compared with the West. Mortality for men and women in Romania is increasing at approximately 6% a year, whereas in the UK there has been a reduction of 1%, and in Belgium the annual reduction in mortality has been 2% over the same time period.

Data regarding the incidence and prevalence of angina (specifically) are much less robust when compared with the mortality data above. Population-based studies show that angina is twice as common in men as in women; that prevalence increases with age (in men aged 45–54 years between 2% and 5%, and 11–20% in age group 65–74 years); and that after the age of 75 years the prevalence is the same in men and women. The prevalence of angina estimated from UK primary care is 1.1% of patients aged between 30 and 59 years, and 2.6% for all ages over 30 years. The number of new cases presenting annually (incidence) varies from 0.44/1000 (age 31–40) to 2.32/1000 (age 61–70) in men, with corresponding numbers for women being 0.08 and 1.01. Fourteen per cent of patients with angina suffered either myocardial infarction or death within 6 months of presentation.[2]

These and other similar data form the basis for interesting speculation as to the causes of IHD which is beyond the scope of this chapter.

Risk factors

The term 'risk factor' in the context of coronary artery disease describes a characteristic (lifestyle, biochemical, physiological or personal) which has been found in observational epidemiological studies to predict the development or presence of atheromatous vascular disease. Lifestyle and biochemical risk factors tend to cluster in an individual, and Framingham Study data demonstrate that the effects of several risk factors are multiplicative rather than additive (particularly cigarette smoking). Patients with clinically established coronary heart disease (such as angina) have for any given risk factor a higher overall level of risk of complications than those without evidence of vascular disease. Because increasing age has a major influence on the absolute frequency of coronary events, the impact of a given risk factor increases with age (up to about 80–85 years old).

The identification of risk factors is important in understanding the pathophysiology of atheroma; in identifying an individual who is at an increased risk of suffering from arterial disease and whose chest pain is therefore more likely to be angina; in improving the prognosis of coronary artery disease in an individual by modifying risk factors; and in reducing the prevalence of IHD in a population by lowering risk factor levels in that population. Of the established risk factors, there are some (age, gender, ethnic origin and family history) which cannot be modified but which may be useful diagnostically; and others which are eminently amenable to change such as cigarette smoking, raised serum cholesterol concentration and high blood pressure. Other risk factors such as obesity and lack of exercise are either less easy to modify or more difficult to prove as being an important risk.

Here follows a list of the more important and established risk factors for atherogenesis and coronary artery disease with a brief commentary on each. Risk factor management is discussed in Chapter 3.

Hypercholesterolaemia

Raised concentration of low-density lipoprotein (LDL) cholesterol is one of the most important risk factors for atheromatous vascular disease, and lowering an individual's serum cholesterol concentration (particularly with a statin) will significantly lower the risk of cardiovascular events. It may be that a raised serum cholesterol concentration is a requirement for atherogenesis, as in Japan, where there is a high rate of cigarette smoking and hypertension, there is a low rate of IHD probably due to the very low serum cholesterol concentrations. However, serum cholesterol concentration taken by itself is a poor predictor of which individual will have a coronary heart disease event.

Low concentration of high density lipoprotein (HDL) cholesterol

HDL cholesterol plays an important part in mobilizing cholesterol from the tissues (reverse transport) and observational studies have shown a higher risk of IHD in those individuals with the lowest concentrations of HDL cholesterol and conversely a protective effect of raised concentrations.

Hypertriglyceridaemia

Because of the problems of the biological variability in fasting triglyceride concentrations, the strong inverse correlation with HDL cholesterol and the association with type 2 diabetes, it has been difficult to establish hypertriglyceridaemia as an independent predictor of coronary risk. Triglycerides (perhaps particularly postprandial levels) may cause atherogenesis by several different mechanisms, but the benefit of specific treatment (rather than attention to the associated metabolic abnormalities) is unclear.

Elevated lipoprotein(a) (Lp(a))

The function of Lp(a) has not been established but it has thrombotic and atherogenic properties and is a major independent determinant of coronary heart disease. However, it cannot be easily and routinely measured, or lowered.

Tobacco use

Cigarette smoking lowers HDL cholesterol

and has a detrimental effect on endothelial function, in addition to increasing platelet aggregation and fibrinogen levels and causing coronary vasospasm. Cigarette smokers have an increased risk of IHD which presents particularly as myocardial infarction and sudden death rather than angina. The risk extends to a lesser degree to non-smokers exposed to cigarette smoke (passive exposure), and to cigar and pipe smokers.

Raised blood pressure

Several observational epidemiological studies in different populations have established a direct relationship between raised blood pressure (both systolic and diastolic) and the incidence of coronary artery disease with no evidence of a threshold level. Raised blood pressure frequently co-exists with other metabolic risk factors (insulin resistance syndrome, metabolic syndrome X).

Diabetes mellitus

Hypertension, obesity and dyslipidaemia frequently accompany diabetes, and hyperinsulinaemia itself may contribute to the development of vascular disease by promoting smooth muscle cell proliferation. Coronary artery disease is a major complication of both type 1 and type 2 diabetes, with relative risk of coronary death of about 2 for men and 3 for women compared with individuals without diabetes, although aggressive control of raised blood pressure and cholesterol may reduce this risk. Atherosclerosis is the cause of death in about 80% of patients with diabetes. The prevalence of diabetes (particularly type 2) is rising such that by year 2010 the world's diabetic population may have doubled, with obvious implications for the prevalence of IHD.

Sex hormones

Case-control and longitudinal studies suggest that women taking combined oral contraceptives have about a threefold increase in the risk of developing IHD, and although the absolute risk is low, it is significantly higher if, in addition, the woman smokes cigarettes. The relative risk of cardiac events is probably lower in postmenopausal women who take oestrogen replacement therapy.

Physical inactivity

Physical inactivity is difficult to quantify and is often associated with other adverse lifestyles, so it is difficult to establish a direct relationship with IHD. In addition, age and obesity are important confounders and many of the intervention studies have recruited subjects post-myocardial infarction. However, several studies have suggested that regular physical activity reduces the risk of coronary events.

Obesity

Being overweight (however defined) is associated with raised concentrations of total cholesterol, triglycerides and blood coagulation factors, raised blood pressure, and an increased risk of diabetes mellitus. The importance of obesity as an independent risk factor may vary with different populations, and may be more significant in men, particularly those with central (abdominal) obesity.

Diet

The relationship between various dietary factors and IHD is potentially very important, as modification of diet may be a relatively inexpensive way of reducing the burden of morbidity from IHD in a population. However, the concept as to what constitutes a 'healthy heart' diet has changed frequently over the years. It is difficult to detach the effects of (say) dietary intake of saturated fats from those of salt, calories (with change in body weight) and fibre, let alone the other variables such as sugar, coffee, antioxidants and the interplay of these and other factors. Manipulation of one aspect of diet often has effects on other aspects, making analysis of effect very difficult. In addition, there are methodological problems (such as dietary recall) encountered in trials of dietary manipulation.

Saturated fat tends to raise and polyunsaturated fat to lower the serum total cholesterol concentration, the latter with potentially beneficial effects. The serum cholesterol concentration of most individuals is derived mainly (about 80%) from hepatic metabolism rather than from dietary cholesterol, so 'low-cholesterol diet' is a misnomer — it is 'cholesterol-lowering' from reduction in saturated fat intake.

Consumption of oily fish lowers serum triglyceride concentration and reduces mortality from IHD. It is not clear whether fish oil supplementation will have a similar effect and whether the beneficial effect is due to modification of blood lipids or to a beneficial effect on endothelial function.

Increased intake of dietary fibre (particularly oat bran and soluble fibre) will reduce serum total cholesterol, and a diet rich in whole grains (brown rice, couscous) reduces rates of IHD.

Haemostatic factors

Elevated fibrinogen levels, reduced fibrinolytic activity and raised coagulation factor VII levels may predict coronary events such as myocardial infarction rather than be predictors of angina and coronary artery disease itself.

Inflammation/infection

Chronic infection causes hyperviscosity by stimulating an acute-phase reaction (which includes hyperfibrinoginaemia), and some organisms may damage the endothelium and predispose to atheroma formation. There is some evidence that chronic infection with *Chlamydia pneumoniae* or *Helicobacter pylori* may be risk factors for atherogenesis and for poorer prognosis in unstable coronary syndromes.

Homocysteine

Elevation of plasma homocysteine has been established as an independent risk factor for coronary, cerebral and peripheral vascular disease, perhaps because it causes endothelial damage. Deficiency of folic acid may contribute to the raised levels, although it is not yet clear whether the increased risk of vascular disease will be modified by folate supplementation.

Alcohol

The effects of alcohol as a risk factor for IHD are difficult to quantify because of the confounding effects of diet, smoking and raised blood pressure in people who drink alcohol, the difficulties of obtaining accurate data on alcohol consumption, and the suggestion that different types of alcoholic drinks may have different protective effects.

However, it seems that moderate alcohol consumption (perhaps up to 3 units daily, i.e. 30 g ethanol) is associated with decreased morbidity and mortality from IHD. The risk reduction may be conveyed through increase in HDL cholesterol concentration, antioxidant levels (flavonoids in red wine) and fibrinolytic activity and inhibition of platelet aggregation.

Personality, stress, psychosocial factors

There is an association between the prevalence of IHD and lower social class and poverty which is probably not entirely explained by the increased number of established risk factors in this population.

Individuals in 'high-demand low-decision' jobs have an increased risk of IHD. Type A behaviour pattern (aggressiveness, ambition, strong sense of time urgency, and abrupt manner of speech and movement) was identified about forty years ago as an independent risk factor for IHD, but later studies have not been able to confirm this. Hostility, mental strain at work, negative life events and lack of social activities independently increase the risk of myocardial infarction.

Low antioxidant activity

The macrophage scavenger receptor recognizes oxidized lipoprotein, and lipid oxidation seems to be a prerequisite for atherogenesis. Increased concentrations of antioxidants may reduce the susceptibility of LDL and Lp(a) cholesterol to oxidation and therefore reduce atherosclerotic risk. Observational studies have demonstrated an inverse relationship between vitamin E intake and IHD events, and vitamin E supplementation has been successful in reducing coronary events post-myocardial infarction. Studies of the effects of dietary supplements with other antioxidants (such as vitamin C) have been less conclusive.

Family history/genotype

A history of IHD before the age of 50 years in a first-degree relative is an independent risk factor.

In addition, familial hypercholesterolaemia and angiotensin-converting enzyme DD genotype are specific genetic risk factors.

Age

IHD increases with increasing age, with a 15-fold increase in men and a 30-fold increase in women from the decade 35–44 to 55–64.

Gender

The incidence of IHD is about five times higher in men up to the age of about 55 years than in women of similar age. The incidence in women increases after the menopause, suggesting a protective effect of female hormones, but in addition women tend to smoke less than men (until recently) and have different distribution of body fat. The onset of symptomatic IHD is about 10 years earlier in men, and only in their ninth decade do women have the same cardiovascular mortality as men.

Race

Ethnic origin itself does not seem to be a major predictor of IHD when environmental factors and other recognized risk factors are taken into account. However, Asian immigrants into the UK seem to form a high-risk group and this increased risk is not adequately explained by the presence of established risk factors, although a metabolic syndrome related to insulin resistance may be relevant.

Clinical history

Heberden introduced the term 'angina pectoris' in a lecture to the Royal College of Physicians of London in 1768 (published in 1772[3]) and in describing the 'sense of strangling and anxiety' suggested that 'angina' was appropriate, as it is derived from *angere*, meaning 'to constrict or choke' (this origin being shared with 'anxious', 'anxiety' and 'anguish'). This classic description includes the sentence 'Those who are affected with it are seized, while they are walking, and more particularly when they walk soon after eating, with a painful and most disagreeable sensation in the breast which seems as if it would take their life away were it to increase or continue: the moment they stand still all this uneasiness vanishes', which well illustrates some of the main features of angina.

The mechanism by which cardiac pain is produced remains poorly understood. However, it is presumed that specific substances (such as adenosine and bradykinin) are released from the myocytes during transient ischaemia and stimulate sensory endings of the intracardiac sympathetic nerves (but specific pain receptors have not been found in the myocardium, although they may exist in coronary arteries), which connect with the upper five thoracic sympathetic ganglia and dorsal root ganglia. Impulses then travel via the spinothalamic tracts and medial pain pathway to the posterior thalamus and thence to the cortex. Vagal fibres connecting to the nucleus of the tractus solitarius and posterior thalamus are also involved. The 'amount' of angina correlates poorly with the severity and duration of myocardial ischaemia (including 'silent' ischaemia) and the central brain connections and affective response may mediate the perception of pain. In addition, somatic awareness (the perception of body activity and physiological functioning) may affect the experience and interpretation of chest discomfort. Angina is visceral (rather than somatic) pain and therefore is poorly localized, difficult to describe and radiates widely in the distribution of the dorsal root ganglia.

A carefully taken clinical history should establish:

- whether symptoms are cardiac in origin and, if so, how limiting are the symptoms; and
- whether symptoms are non-cardiac in origin and there is an alternative diagnosis.

Chest pain

It is assumed that the 'central, crushing, substernal ache with radiation to the left arm' is well known and appreciated as being suggestive of angina, so what follows is an attempt to highlight some of the lesser known features of ischaemic heart pain.

Character

Although the symptom is described as 'chest pain', patients rarely use the word 'pain' and often deny that pain is the problem, using words such as 'discomfort', 'heaviness', 'tightness' and 'pressure'. Anxiety, breathlessness and sweating may accompany the symptoms and the discomfort gradually builds up over a period of a minute or so (sudden onset suggests thoracic aortic dissection or pulmonary embolus). The pain may be described as 'burning', raising the obvious possibility of gastro-oesophageal origin, and there is evidence to suggest that acid reflux may cause oesophageal pain and coronary artery spasm leading to cardiac pain.

Pain which is described as 'sharp', 'stabbing' or 'knife-like' is rarely cardiac in origin. It is worth observing the patient's hands when the symptoms are described. Fingers curled into a clenched fist over the upper part of the sternum (Levine's sign) suggests cardiac pain. Angina may present without 'pain', but with 'angina equivalents' such as breathlessness, faintness or burping, and these atypical symptoms tend to be more common in the elderly and in patients with diabetes.

Although the character of symptoms described above varies from one patient to another, an individual tends to experience the same symptoms throughout the natural history of the condition. It is very useful, therefore, to ask a patient who has had angina previously documented whether the present symptoms are similar. However, pain pathways may become facilitated by chronic pain so that cardiac symptoms take on the character of cervical root pain if, for example, a patient subsequently suffers from prolapsed cervical intervertebral disc.

Location and radiation

The discomfort is typically retrosternal but may be felt anywhere from mandible to xiphisternum (and rarely outside this area — maxilla and epigastrium). Radiation is to both shoulders and arms as far as the fingertips (more commonly the left), and sensation may be felt only in one of these areas ('arm heaviness', for example). Less frequently there is radiation through to the back, but any pain which is described as 'between the shoulder blades' should be considered initially to be due to thoracic aortic dissection (or musculoskeletal).

It is useful to ask patients the 'size' of their pain and to demonstrate it with their hand. An area the size of one or two fingers is not angina, particularly if the finger points over the apex of the heart. Similarly, angina is felt in only one location and does not flit from one area to another.

Duration

Most episodes of angina last between 1 and 5 min (very rarely longer than 20 min) and not seconds (less than 5) or many hours.

Cardiac pain lasting longer than about 30 min (in the absence of non-sinus tachycardia) should be considered to be due to myocardial infarction, although there is a fine line to be drawn between 'severe angina' and 'small myocardial infarction' in terms of loss of heart muscle.

Provoking and relieving factors

Any condition that reduces myocardial oxygen delivery or increases oxygen consumption may cause angina.

The typical precipitant is walking, particularly up an incline and when carrying a heavy bag in one hand. It may be the effect of handgrip when carrying (which causes hypertensive and chronotropic stress on the heart) rather than the additional work which exacerbates angina. Angina may be felt at lower work rate when walking into a cold wind — the cold causes coronary artery vasoconstriction, and moving cool air over the 'snout area' causes a systemic hypertensive response (angina can be reduced by covering the nose and mouth with a scarf in addition to wearing warm clothing) — or after a meal (increase in splanchnic bloodflow and consequently cardiac output in response to digestion).

Even when all these are taken into account, the reproducibility of the exercise stress which causes angina is low — there are some times when angina seems to be caused by relatively little exercise and vice versa. The severity of coronary arterial disease, the capacity for vasodilatation, the extent of collateral vessel development and

the health of the myocardium will all contribute to this variability but in addition part of the explanation may be 'first effort', 'walk through' or 'warm-up' (or occasionally 'first hole') angina. This occurs in some people when they develop angina with exertion, stop and are then able to continue at the same level of exertion without developing symptoms. Angina is often precipitated early in the day by relatively little physical activity, whereas later more vigorous exertion is required. This phenomenon may be due to ischaemic preconditioning in which brief periods of myocardial ischaemia with intermittent reperfusion protect against a subsequent (and perhaps longer) ischaemic insult. The mechanism is unknown but may involve an increase in the activity of antioxidant and heat-shock proteins which will protect against damage caused by free radicals.[4]

Other provoking factors include emotion (often anger, frustration or excitement).

Angina which wakes the patient from sleep may be associated with dreaming or with coronary artery spasm, perhaps precipitated by gastro-oesophageal reflux.

If there appears to be no provoking factor, paroxysmal tachycardia, particularly atrial fibrillation, may be the cause.

Not infrequently, angina is caused by a combination of several of these precipitants and tends to be more common in the morning. Thus a typical history is of angina occurring shortly after leaving the house in the morning after breakfast during a brisk walk to work heading into a cold wind and carrying a briefcase.

Angina is relieved by abolishing the precipitating factor. This usually means stopping exercise. It is possible to slow the heart by carotid massage and the strain phase of Valsalva manoeuvre, but this is rarely recommended.

Relief may be hastened by the use of sublingual trinitrin (usually in the form of a spray) and this forms the basis of a diagnostic therapeutic trial. Discomfort should be relieved within a maximum of about 3 min but pain due to gastro-oesophageal spasm may also be helped. (A better therapeutic trial to distinguish oesophageal from cardiac pain is to use a proton pump inhibitor given for 2 weeks in maximum dose.)

Exertional angina should be helped by beta-blocker, and coronary artery spasm by either nitrate or calcium channel antagonist.

Patients should be warned against lying down when they have angina because the increase in venous return increases cardiac work and ventricular dimensions and exacerbates myocardial ischaemia (decubitus angina).

Chest discomfort which increases with inspiration, local chest pressure or arm movement is unlikely to be due to angina, but repeated arm movements (such as cleaning a window) increase oxygen consumption more than the same amount of work done by leg muscles and may precipitate myocardial ischaemia.

Associated symptoms
Breathlessness

Heberden described patients with angina as having 'no shortness of breath', but dyspnoea may be a feature of myocardial ischaemia. Regional impairment of left ventricular function is an early manifestation of ischaemia (while pain is a late and inconsistent feature), and if the area of ischaemia is large or the function of the remainder of the ventricle is chronically impaired, then acute left ventricular failure may ensue and cause breathlessness. Also, patients will vary in their description of ischaemic heart pain, with some interpreting the sensation of tightness as shortness of breath, particularly if it limits exercise; and patients who have 'painless ischaemia' (the elderly and those with diabetes mellitus) will tend to have dyspnoea as the presenting symptom of angina.

Sweating

Reflex sympathetic stimulation accompanies the fall in cardiac output which may follow myocardial ischaemia, causing tachycardia, sweating and cutaneous vasoconstriction.

Syncope

Loss of consciousness is not a feature of uncomplicated angina, although it may rarely occur when myocardial ischaemia causes transient reduction in cardiac output in patients with severely compromised left ventricular function. Otherwise, syncope is due to atrioventricular block, sinus node arrest or a pulseless tachyarrhythmia (particularly self-terminating ventricular fibrillation) associated with ischaemia.

Perhaps the most common cause of syncope is the hypotension caused by self-administration of sublingual nitrate taken to relieve the attack of angina. Nitrate causes venodilatation and pooling of blood in the periphery which leads to a fall in venous return to the heart at a time when the myocardium is recovering from the effects of ischaemia. The consequent fall in cardiac output and systemic hypotension may lead to syncope, particularly if the patient has recently assumed the standing position, consumed alcohol and is in a warm atmosphere. Patients should be advised to sit prior to taking sublingual trinitrin and for 10 min afterwards.

Fatigue

Reduction in cardiac output caused by myocardial ischaemia may lead to muscle fatigue which may be noted on exertion and present as a prominent symptom. More frequently, patients will say that a severe episode of angina 'knocks them out' for a variable length of time. The mechanism is not known but anxiety is likely to play a large part.

Those of underlying disorder

Examples are weight loss from thyroid overactivity, tendinitis associated with hypercholesterolaemia and post-exertional syncope of aortic stenosis.

There may also be symptomatic evidence of the non-cardiac effects of atherosclerosis, such as intermittent claudication, past history of stroke or transient cerebral ischaemia

Assessment

The aim of assessment is to document the severity of the symptoms and stratify risk.

The severity of angina is suggested by the degree of restriction of activity and modification of lifestyle which the patient has to endure. The frequency of angina and the precipitating events are considered, remembering that reduced frequency of attacks may reflect the patient 'slowing down' to prevent symptoms rather than improvement of the underlying condition. In addition, limitation may arise from respiratory or locomotor disease rather than angina.

There are several grading classifications of angina, each based on activity scale or status, but for usual clinical activity (rather than research) it is better to document the specific activity which precipitates discomfort tailored to the individual (walking 100 m on flat ground, walking across a ploughed field carrying a shotgun, etc.).

Patients must not drive cars or motorcycles if angina occurs at rest or when they are driving, but they may resume when symptoms are controlled, and the drivers' licensing authority (DVLA) need not be notified. However, patients who are holders of a group 2 entitlement (large lorries and buses, and medium-sized goods vehicles and minibuses) must notify the DVLA, and their license will be revoked until they are free of symptoms for at least 6 weeks and can meet the exercise requirements.

Assessment for risk stratification aims to identify patients with angina who are at increased risk of death or myocardial infarction and who require urgent investigation and treatment. This, in essence, involves distinguishing patients with chronic stable angina from those with unstable angina. The former has a relatively good prognosis, with an annual mortality of approximately 2–3% and a further similar percentage each year suffering from non-fatal myocardial infarction. The increasingly widespread use of lipid-lowering treatment for secondary prevention may well reduce these percentages. In addition, there is a group of patients with chronic stable angina whose prognosis will be improved by revascularization (impairment of left ventricular function, multiple vessel disease, proximal stenoses) and who may be identified by the severity of their symptoms but who will often require investigation (such as objective evidence of exercise performance).

Patients with new presentation of angina (less than 6 months) are at increased risk of myocardial infarction or death (14% in one study[5]), as are those who have unstable angina.

Unstable angina

This is defined by one of the following three features in the absence of evidence of acute myocardial infarction:

- stable, exertional angina pectoris in which symptoms become increasingly severe, prolonged or frequent;
- angina of new onset which is precipitated by minimal exertion;
- angina which occurs at rest (other than Prinzmetal's variant angina).

Patients are often aware of a change in the pattern of their symptoms. The quality of the discomfort is the same but tends to be more intense, may last for up to 30 min and may occur at rest or at night. There may be radiation to a different site and also new associated features such as sweating, breathlessness or nausea. Rest and sublingual trinitrin give only temporary or incomplete relief.

Unstable angina is of particular concern when episodes occur at rest or without any precipitating factors, and when it occurs within 2 weeks of acute myocardial infarction. It is always worth remembering that there may be an 'extrinsic' cause such as anaemia, infection, fever, hyperthyroidism or tachycardia (secondary unstable angina).

The concern is that unstable angina will progress to myocardial infarction. The great majority will not, however, progress in the short term (particularly with treatment), but over half will suffer an adverse cardiac event in the subsequent 8 months. Patients with unstable angina require identification and immediate (or within 7 days depending on the clinical picture) referral for specialist assessment, treatment and investigation.[2]

Examination

The physical examination of patients with angina is usually normal but may show:

- evidence of acute myocardial ischaemia during an attack — third or fourth heart sound, mitral systolic murmur, hypotension;
- evidence of chronic myocardial ischaemia — heart failure, dyskinetic ventricular impulse;
- conditions which cause or contribute to angina, such as anaemia, thyroid overactivity, vasculitis, valvular heart disease, hypertrophic cardiomyopathy, atrial fibrillation with uncontrolled ventricular response, nicotine staining of the fingers or hair;
- evidence of non-cardiac atheromatous vascular disease such as peripheral vascular disease, stroke;
- hypertension with or without clinical evidence of hypertensive end-organ damage;
- features of hyperlipidaemia;
- subclinical evidence of vascular disease such as low ankle brachial pressure index;
- transverse earlobe crease. There is a statistical association between a deep diagonal crease of the earlobes and coronary artery disease (not found in Japanese or Chinese populations).
- another condition which may account for chest pain — hyperventilation, chest wall tenderness (particularly over the costochondral junctions — Tietze described tender swelling of the costochondral junctions, which is very uncommon), mitral valve prolapse

(Barlow's syndrome), right upper quadrant tenderness associated with gallbladder disease.

What is often required from the history and examination of a patient whose complaint is of 'chest pain' is an answer to the question 'is the pain cardiac in origin?'. If the pain is non-cardiac, then there may be an alternative specific diagnosis or one of 'chest pain? cause'. The diagnosis of cardiac pain in the outpatient department has important implications for the patient and his management, but there is an additional major impact on resource allocation in the diagnosis of patients presenting to the emergency services where the decision to advise hospital admission is often based on the clinical history, usually with additional information from an electrocardiogram. A study from Manchester, UK[6] objectively assessed the usefulness of aspects of a structured history in the distinction of cardiac from non-cardiac pain. The pain was more likely to be cardiac if:

- the patient was older (but there was no effect of gender);
- the chest pain was central and described as 'heavy';
- there was radiation to the arms;
- the pain was similar to a previous episode ascribed to angina;
- exercise made the pain worse;

- the pain was relieved by nitrates.

The pain was less likely to be cardiac if it was submammary and exacerbated by deep breaths and hunger, and relief by rest or antacids and the association with sweating, palpitation and breathlessness was not helpful. Using this structured history and with a normal electrocardiogram on admission and the following morning, the authors were able to identify within 24 h patients whose chest pain was of cardiac origin with a sensitivity of 98% and specificity of 95%. This study is an example of the way in which a careful history which incorporates elements of the features described in this chapter helps to identify patients whose symptoms are angina.

References

1. Sans S, Kesteloot H, Kromhout D, on behalf of the Task Force of the European Society of Cardiology on Cardiovascular Mortality and Morbidity Statistics in Europe, *Eur Heart J* 1997; **18**: 1231–48.

2. DeBono D, Hopkins A, on behalf of the working party of the Joint Audit Committee of the British Cardiac Society and the Royal College of Physicians of London, Guidelines. Investigation and management of stable angina, *J R Coll Physicians Lond* 1993; **27**: 267–73.

3. Heberden W, Some account of a disorder of the breast, *Med Trans R Coll Physicians Lond* 1772; **2**: 59.

4. Yellon DM, Baxter GF, Marber MS, Angina

reassessed: pain or protector? *Lancet* 1996; **347**: 1159–62.

5. Duncan B, Fulton M, Morison SL et al, Prognosis of new and worsening angina pectoris, *Br Med J* 1976; **1**: 891–985.

6. Millane T, Hearing SD, Jones PE, Brooks NH, Two ECGs and a history: a guide to early hospital discharge of patients with 'chest pain? cause', *J R Coll Physicians Lond* 1998; **32**: 122–4.

Non-invasive investigations

Martin R Bennett

2

Introduction

The purpose of non-invasive investigation for suspected angina is several-fold:

1. to establish that the patient presenting with chest pain has ischaemic heart disease;
2. to indicate which region(s) of the left ventricular wall is/are affected;
3. to estimate the severity of the ischaemic heart disease (the ischaemic burden);
4. the evaluation of recoverable myocardium after coronary angioplasty or bypass grafting.

Non-invasive investigations all rely on the comparison of an investigation undertaken when the heart is under 'stress', usually exercise- or drug-induced tachycardia, and a similar investigation in the basal or resting state. When a segment of myocardium becomes ischaemic, there is a cascade of physiological events with increasing ischaemia. Thus, the earliest event is a perfusion defect in the affected segment, followed in order by regional diastolic dysfunction, regional systolic dysfunction, global left ventricular (LV) dysfunction, ischaemic ST segment depression, and, finally, the development of angina.[1] Treadmill testing relies on changes in ECG characteristics and haemodynamic parameters such as heart rate and blood pressure. Nuclear scans rely on changes in myocardial uptake of tracers (as a measure of myocardial perfusion), and stress echocardiography relies upon the development of regional wall motion abnormalities in segments of the LV cavity which develop as a result of ischaemia. None of the investigations are 100% accurate, and their accuracy is defined by their sensitivity, the ability to detect a true diagnosis when the disease is present (estimated as the ratio of true positives/total number of patients with coronary artery disease (CAD)), and their specificity, their ability to reject the diagnosis when it is absent (estimated as true negatives/total number of patients without CAD). The criteria for positivity of any of the tests is a compromise between the highest sensitivity, so that patients with disease are not missed, with high specificity, so that not too many patients are misdiagnosed or mis-investigated. In general, the more stringent the diagnostic criteria, the higher the specificity, but the lower the sensitivity. A further measure, the predictive value of the test, is the likelihood that the individual with a positive test has CAD (estimated as the true positives/total number of positives). The predictive value (unlike the sensitivity and specificity) is very much affected by the prevalence of the disease in the population under study, and dramatically falls with a low incidence of CAD. In many cases the tests provide similar, but complementary, evidence of myocardial ischaemia. However, each has its own specific niche in the investigation of the patient with suspected or proven ischaemic heart disease.

Exercise electrocardiography (treadmill testing)

Exercise electrocardiography is widely used in the diagnosis of CAD. In patients with suspected CAD, exercise testing may confirm the diagnosis and indicate the severity and prognosis of the disease, although there are too many false-positive results to advocate its widespread use as a screen for asymptomatic CAD. Exercise testing can be used to follow patients with known CAD, including the outcome of therapeutic interventions such as drug treatment or revascularization. Exercise testing can also be used to risk stratify patients post myocardial infarction.

Contraindications to exercise testing

These are listed in Table 2.1. However, it should also be noted that a number of conditions cause resting ST segment changes, which make

Table 2.1
Contraindications to stress testing.

Acute myocardial infarction (early, within 7 days)
Unstable angina
Congestive cardiac failure on clinical criteria
Acute myocarditis/endocarditis
Left ventricular outflow obstruction/hypertrophic cardiomyopathy
Severe aortic or mitral stenosis
Severe tachyarrhythmias
Dissecting aortic aneurysm
Left main stem stenosis

interpretation of the exercise ECG either difficult or impossible (see below), when other forms of non-invasive imaging are preferable.

Protocol

Exercise electrocardiography is usually performed with a standardized protocol of graded exercise, usually performed on a bicycle ergometer or motorized treadmill. One of the commonest is the Bruce protocol,[2] which is widely applicable to a variety of patients (Table 2.2). A modified version, or a protocol outlined by Naughton, can be used for patients with known cardiorespiratory disease, or inability to exercise vigorously for other reasons. The patient undergoes uninterrupted exercise to a graded protocol,

and the test is terminated at a defined endpoint. This is frequently once a target heart rate has been reached (usually at 220 beats minus age in years, or 85% of this for a modified protocol). Alternatively, the test can be terminated for a variety of other reasons (Table 2.3). Heart rate and ECG are monitored continuously, blood pressure every 2–3 min, and monitoring is continued immediately after exercise, 3 min into recovery and at subsequent 2–3-min intervals until the ECG has normalized.

Interpretation of exercise electrocardiographs

There are a number of ECG abnormalities which are classified as criteria for positive tests.

Table 2.2
The Bruce protocol for exercise testing.

Stage	Speed (miles/h)	Grade (%)	Duration (min)
0[a]	1.7	0	–
1/2[a]	1.7	5	–
1[b]	1.7	10	3
2	2.5	12	3
3	3.4	14	3
4	4.2	16	3
5	5.0	18	3
6	5.5	20	3
7	6.0	22	3

[a] Indicates stages in the modified Bruce protocol.
[b] Indicates the start of the full Bruce protocol.

Table 2.3
Indications for termination of stress testing.

Target heart rate achieved

Severe angina and/or ST segment depression >2 mm

Severe hypertension (SBP >250 mmHg or diastolic >110 mmHg)

Severe hypotension (>20 mmHg drop on exercise)

Severe arrhythmias/symptomatic bradycardia

Severe non-cardiac problems (e.g. dyspnoea, claudication)

Patient's demand

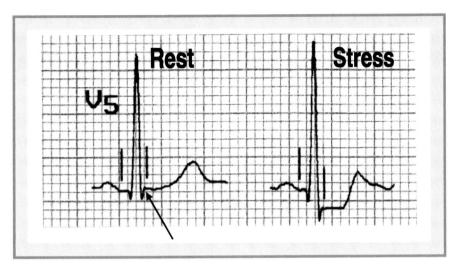

Figure 2.1
Assesssment of ST depression is performed 0.08 s past the J point (arrow) of the ECG.

The ST segments may be horizontally depressed, up- or down-sloping, although depression of the J point of the QRS complex without significant ST depression is a normal response to exercise. The most widely used definition of a positive test is the development of >1 mm ST horizontal or down-sloping ST depression 0.08 s after the J point (Figs 2.1 and 2.2).

Exercise electrocardiography is a rapid method of screening for CAD in groups of patients with a moderately high risk of having such disease. However, its false-positive rates are too high to recommend its use in low-risk populations.[3,4] Meta-analyses of the diagnostic efficiency of exercise electrocardiography indicate a sensitivity of 81% but a specificity of only 66% in the diagnosis of multivessel coronary disease.[5] A study from the same group, increasing the number of patients included, returned figures of 68% and 77% respectively,[6] although these figures are better for the diagnosis of any coronary disease. There are a number of causes of ST depression during exercise (Table 2.4) which contribute to the poor predictive value of exercise testing, but many confounding factors are unknown.

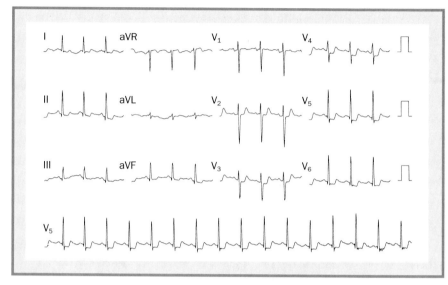

Figure 2.2
A 'positive' exercise ECG, showing >2 mm horizontal ST segment depression at peak exercise in V4–V5.

In general, the sensitivity of exercise testing depends upon a number of factors. In particular, sensitivity is much reduced when submaximal testing is used, or when beta-blockade is used, often requiring repeat testing having not used this therapy on the day of the test. False negatives are also often encountered with ischaemia in territory supplied by the left circumflex artery, which is often electrically silent.

Special indications for exercise electrocardiography

Post-myocardial infarction

The purpose of exercise electrocardiography after myocardial infarction (MI) is to identify patients at high risk of subsequent infarction or death. The test is often performed just prior to discharge, or 4–6 weeks later, and is usually symptom-limited or submaximal (see above). However, there is considerable controversy over the prognostic value of

Table 2.4
Causes of ST segment depression on exercise electrocardiography other than ischaemia.

Abnormal resting ECG	*Previous MI*
	Bundle branch block
	Pre-excitation
Ventricular hypertrophy	*Systemic hypertension*
	Pulmonary hypertension
	Aortic stenosis
	Pulmonary stenosis
Cardiomyopathy	*Hypertrophic cardiomyopathy*
	Dilated cardiomyopathy
Drugs	*Digoxin and other anti-arrhythmics*
Other	*Females*
	Smoking or food prior to exercise
	Mitral valve prolapse

testing, especially if focused on ST segment changes alone. Some studies have claimed that exercise testing can identify a subgroup of patients >10 times more likely to die in the first year after MI.[7] Other studies indicate that there is no prognostic value of a positive test on ECG criteria alone,[8-10] although the test does identify patients who are more likely to develop angina. However, the development of ventricular arrhythmia or a poor haemodynamic response to exercise significantly improves the predictive value of exercise ECGs in identifying patients at risk of sudden death.[8]

Nuclear scans

Nuclear scans for the detection of ischaemic heart disease rely upon the detection of differences between distribution of a radiolabelled contrast agent in ischaemic and non-ischaemic segments of the left ventricle. Thus, the label is delivered at peak stress, either exercise or pharmacological stress, and images are compared at peak stress, and a few hours or days later, under resting conditions.

Choice of agents used

The commonest contrast agents used for nuclear scanning are thallium-201 (Tl) or technetium-99m (Tc), as either ^{99m}Tc sestamibi (MIBI) or ^{99m}Tc tetrofosmin. Tl is a metallic element which behaves similarly to potassium, with a high intracellular concentration. Approximately 88% of Tl is cleared from the blood with the first circulation after intravenous injection, with peak myocardial uptake at about 10 min after injection.[11] ^{201}Tl has a number of limitations, in particular a low photon energy leading to low resolution images and significant attenuation by soft tissue shadows. In addition, only 4% of the label is retained by the myocardium, with the rest accumulating mainly in skeletal muscle and gut, producing high background counts. For these reasons, together with an undesirably long half-life, ^{201}Tl has largely been replaced by ^{99m}Tc in many centres for routine perfusion scanning. In contrast to ^{201}Tl, ^{99m}Tc as sestamibi or tetrofosmin conjugates are lipophilic, and myocardial distribution is proportional to bloodflow. Cardiac uptake and retention depends upon mitochondrial function, so that uptake is reduced and washout increased by severe ischaemia. In contrast, ^{201}Tl redistribution with stress represents heterogeneous bloodflow rather than ischaemia.[12] Clearance from the blood of ^{99m}Tc conjugates is rapid, with half-lives of 2–5 min, with better retention of tracer in the myocardium compared with ^{201}Tl.[13]

Protocols

The different retention characteristics of ^{201}Tl and ^{99m}Tc mean that different imaging protocols are required for each agent. ^{201}Tl is retained in the heart with an elimination half-life of approximately 7 h. ^{201}Tl is therefore given at peak stress, and continued for 2 min to obtain stable conditions for tracer extraction, and stress images are obtained within 5–30 min of administration. The slow equilibration of intracellular and intravascular ^{201}Tl means that redistribution within the myocardium occurs over several hours, so that images obtained 3–4 h later are similar to those which would be obtained at rest, and no separate resting injection is required.

In contrast, redistribution of ^{99m}Tc conjugates is low (<15%), which allows stress images to be obtained up to 4 h after injection. However, this lack of redistribution means that separate stress and rest injections need to be given, and the 6-h half-life of ^{99m}Tc means that, ideally, injections should be performed on separate days for ^{99m}Tc sestamibi, although the slightly faster clearance of ^{99}Tc tetrofosmin means that a 1-day protocol is adequate. The choice of 1- or 2-day protocols will obviously also depend upon local factors, such as the availability of imaging equipment and staff, and patient demographics.[14] However, for imaging purposes, the 2-day protocol is preferred, as it is more reliable, has smaller quantities of residual activity, has a lower radiation burden, and allows the doctor to intervene if the stress images are conclusively normal.

Detection of ischaemic segments

Uptake in the redistribution images reflects the amount of muscle present, while the stress images reflect both the muscle mass and stress perfusion. With ²⁰¹Tl, normal myocardium appears as an area of high uptake during stress, but with rapid washout. Reversible ischaemia appears as an area with defects on stress images, which improves on the redistribution images (Fig. 2.3). In contrast, an infarcted region appears as a defect in both stress and rest images, and mixed patterns of reversible and fixed defects are common, particularly in the era of thrombolysis. Severe ischaemia is also demonstrated by very slow redistribution, with reduction in resting perfusion. This is the basis of the use of ²⁰¹Tl in the detection of hibernating myocardium (see below). The identification of reversibly ischaemic, infarcted or normal segments on ⁹⁹ᵐTc imaging is similar to that for ²⁰¹Tl imaging.

Other appearances on nuclear scanning can also indicate ischaemia. For example, dilatation of the ventricular cavity on stress which resolves with exercise implies extensive reversible ischaemia and carries a poor

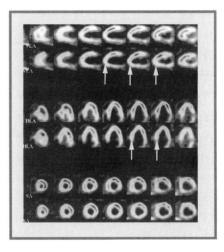

Figure 2.3
⁹⁹Tc MIBI scan at rest (upper) and stress (lower), indicating higher bloodflow in segments at rest (arrows). Images are vertical long axis (VLA) displayed septum to lateral, horizontal short axis (HLA) displayed anterior to inferior, and short axis (SA) displayed apex to base.

prognosis.[15] In contrast, the significance of reversed defects, which are more apparent at rest than on exercise, is uncertain, although such a pattern can arise in the presence of partial infarction with a patent coronary artery.[16]

Artefacts and limitations of nuclear scans

Nuclear scans of myocardial perfusion have a number of limitations for the detection of

Table 2.5
Diseases other than coronary artery disease resulting in perfusion defects on nuclear scans.

Dynamic coronary obstruction	Coronary artery spasm Muscle bridging Syndrome X
Small vessel disease	Diabetes mellitus
Anomalous coronary arteries	
Intrinsic muscle disease	Hypertrophic cardiomyopathy Dilated cardiomyopathy Ventricular hypertrophy
Infiltrative cardiac disease	Amyloid
	Sarcoid
	Connective tissue disease
Left bundle branch block	

ischaemia, and anatomical factors should be considered when interpreting scans, to allow for normal attenuation of a number of regions of the left ventricular wall. In particular, the inferior wall is attenuated by being further from the camera and more prone to artefacts resulting from respiratory movement. The anterior wall can be attenuated by breast shadows and the apical segment or basal septum, because these are the thinnest sections of the ventricular wall. Perfusion defects are also apparent in a number of cardiac diseases other than CAD (Table 2.5), some of which are reversible on redistribution images.

Most of the potential sources of artefact on nuclear scanning are obvious, but left bundle branch block merits further comment. Left bundle branch block is one of the commonest reasons for requesting nuclear scans, because the stress ECG cannot be interpreted. However, in left bundle branch block, delayed relaxation shortens the duration of diastolic bloodflow in the septum. This results in inadequate coronary flow during tachycardia[17] and can produce reversible perfusion defects in the absence of CAD. This is more likely with defects identified in the anterior or septal regions. If tachycardia is kept to a minimum by using pharmacological stress rather than exercise, then the false positives are reduced.[18] However, it should also be noted that the commonest cause of reversible perfusion defects in patients with left bundle branch block is CAD.[19]

Predictive power of nuclear scans

Meta-analysis review of nuclear perfusion scanning with exercise stress indicates a sensitivity and specificity of 84% and 87% (for planar scans) or 96% and 83% for tomography, when angiography is used as the gold standard.[20] Pharmacological stress agents such as dipyridamole or adenosine return a sensitivity/specificity of 87%/74% and 87%/88% respectively compared with angiography,[21,22] and there is a good agreement between either dipyridamole or adenosine nuclear scans and those obtained by exercise.[21,22] Both sensitivity and specificity are reduced considerably with submaximal stress, and a low threshold should therefore be used for pharmacological stress testing rather than exercise in patients with impaired exercise capacity or motivation.

When compared with exercise electrocardiography (treadmill testing),

nuclear scanning appears much superior in determining the presence of CAD.[23] This is probably not surprising, considering that perfusion defects are the earliest detectable changes in the myocardium upon ischaemia.[1] Nuclear scanning also gives good information regarding the localization of ischaemia compared with exercise electrocardiography, which is particularly poor in this regard.[24]

Nuclear scanning is also a very accurate indicator of future coronary events. Normal ^{201}Tl imaging is associated with a cardiac event rate (cardiac death, myocardial infarction) of 0.5–1%/year, which was similar to that observed in the general population under study.[25–27] The presence of markedly abnormal exercise electrocardiography does not increase the event rate of patients with normal thallium tests, indicating the superiority of nuclear scanning compared with exercise ECGs. This means that perfusion scanning can be used to identify a very low risk group of patients who may not require coronary angiography. The overall prognostic power of abnormal nuclear scans to detect high-risk patients depends upon the abnormality found on the nuclear scan, but adverse predictors of prognosis include increased lung uptake of thallium (related to LV dysfunction), LV dilatation at rest or with stress, the extent and severity of the perfusion defect, and the presence of redistribution or a multi-territory abnormality. In general, thallium scanning has a prognostic power similar to or slightly superior to that of coronary angiography, but very much superior to exercise electrocardiography. Exercise and pharmacological stress and thallium imaging have similar abilities to predict adverse cardiac events.

Specific indications for nuclear scans

Hibernation

Hibernation can be defined as contractile dysfunction present at rest which is reversible with revascularization. It appears to be due to reduced resting myocardial perfusion, although it is associated with the loss of contractile proteins and glycogen accumulation in the long term. The identification of hibernation is important, as resting ventricular function is closely related to prognosis, and improvement in left ventricular function following revascularization in patients with hibernating myocardium can improve both symptoms and prognosis.[28,29] In addition, the identification of significant hibernation may allow a patient to undergo conventional revascularization rather than transplantation.

The detection of hibernating myocardium can be achieved by both positron emission tomography (PET) and conventional nuclear

cardiology using ^{201}Tl or ^{99m}Tc. Normal myocardium preferentially uses fatty acids for its metabolic demands, but hibernating myocardium switches to the utilization of glucose uptake. Thus, uptake of a metabolic tracer such as fluorine ^{18}deoxyglucose (^{18}F-FDG) is high in hibernating versus normal myocardium. The combined use of a tracer analysing blood flow, such as ^{13}N-ammonia or ^{15}O-water, confirms that the hibernating segments also have impaired regional blood flow. The detection of the metabolic changes by PET scanning makes this technique the gold standard for detecting hibernation.[30] However, the limited availability of the technology and the expense mean that conventional nuclear cardiology tracers also have a role.

The use of ^{201}Tl or ^{99m}Tc tracers to detect hibernation relies upon demonstrating a mismatch between contractile function and myocardial mass in the same segments. The contractile dysfunction is usually detected with high-resolution anatomical techniques, such as echocardiography or magnetic resonance imaging. The maximum tracer uptake, which reflects muscle mass, is then identified using ^{201}Tl or ^{99m}Tc. There are considerable differences in the protocols used for acquiring the perfusion images, reflecting a lack of consensus on the optimal mode of acquisition. In general, stress and rest perfusion is obtained during the appropriate

Table 2.6
Indications for pharmacological echocardiography.

Patient unable to exercise
Non-diagnostic exercise test
Investigation of ischaemia pre- and post-revascularization in known ischaemic heart disease patients
Investigation of viable myocardium pre-revascularization
Risk stratification before surgery or after myocardial infarction

times, and the best muscle mass obtained after the fullest redistribution of the rest image. Hibernation can be seen as impaired segmental contraction with reduced rest perfusion images, which become near-normal rest-redistribution images.

Left ventricular dysfunction

Normally, 5–15% of the administered ^{201}Tl is taken up by the lungs. In left ventricular failure, with a rise in capillary wedge pressure, uptake may be significantly greater and may even occur at rest. This has been found to be a prognostically important indicator of severity of left ventricular dysfunction.

Stress echocardiography

At rest, infarcted areas of the left ventricular wall are visualized as hypokinetic or akinetic segments on echocardiography. In contrast, areas which are adequately perfused at rest but become ischaemic on exercise contract normally at rest, but develop segmental wall motion abnormalities on exercise or after pharmacological stress. Stress is usually provided as a graded exercise, similar to treadmill testing, or as either a vasodilator (adenosine, dipyridamole) or inotropic agent (dobutamine, arbutamine, isoprenaline).

Choice of stress agent

In general, exercise is the preferred stress agent for echocardiography in patients who can exercise. This is because exercise provides a more physiological stress and the double product (HR $\times$ SBP) is greater.[31] This means that exercise echocardiography can produce a higher ischaemic burden, and that pharmacological stress may underestimate the

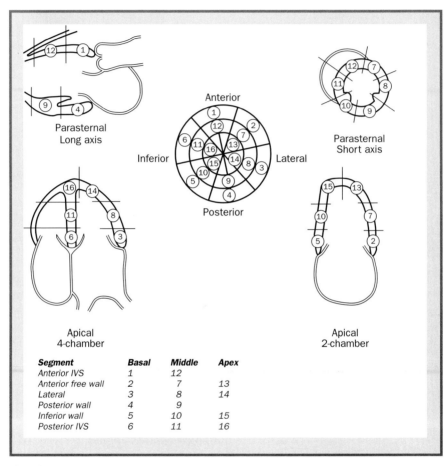

Figure 2.4
Division of the left ventricular wall into segments for stress echocardiographic assessment.

Segment	Basal	Middle	Apex
Anterior IVS	1	12	
Anterior free wall	2	7	13
Lateral	3	8	14
Posterior wall	4	9	
Inferior wall	5	10	15
Posterior IVS	6	11	16

severity of ischaemia.[32] This means that pharmacological stress should only be used for specific indications (Table 2.6). The contraindications for stress echocardiography are similar to those for exercise electrocardiography. However, exercise echocardiography also has limitations, in particular the inability to obtain images

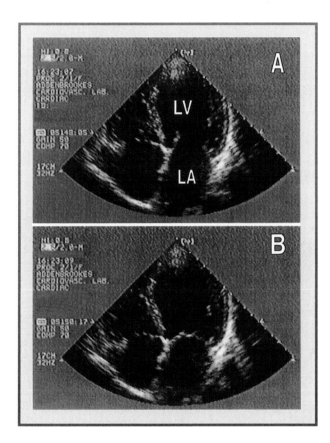

Figure 2.5
Long axis stress
echocardiographic images of
(A) diastolic and (B) systolic
frames at peak stress,
showing stress-induced LV
dilatation, and extensive wall
motion abnormalities. LV,
left ventricle, LA, left atrium.

during the exercise test, and a high respiratory rate at peak exercise precluding optimal imaging. Comparison of exercise versus dobutamine echocardiography has shown similar sensitivities for both methods (63–75% for one vessel disease, 80–90% for two-vessel disease, and 100% for three-vessel disease) and specificity of 87% for both methods.[33]

Protocol

Protocols for stress echocardiography obviously vary between institutions and

Table 2.7
Causes of segmental wall motion abnormalities other than ischaemia.

Left bundle branch block
Permanent pacemaker insertion
Post cardiac surgery
Wolff–Parkinson–White syndrome
Focal intrinsic cardiac muscle disease (myocarditis, sarcoid, etc.)
Right ventricular volume/pressure overload
Aortic regurgitation

according to the stress agent, either exercise or pharmacological. In general, the patient is studied in the left decubitus position, with a 12-lead ECG monitor attached, with recordings taken at each stage and during recovery. Heart rate and blood pressure are recorded at each stage of the protocol, with full resuscitation equipment available. In general, the reasons for termination of a stress echo study are the same as for stress electrocardiography. However, the development of LV outflow obstruction as assessed on Doppler imaging should be added. It should also be noted that a systolic drop of >20 mmHg from resting values or >10 mmHg from previous values during dobutamine echocardiography is not associated with LV dysfunction, a marker of severity of ischaemic heart disease, or associated with a poor prognosis.[34,35] Indeed, a hypotensive response may occur in 5–20% of patients.[34,35]

The heart is visualized echocardiographically in the standard parasternal long and short axis and the apical four- and two-chamber views. Images are generally acquired at rest, at peak stress, and during recovery. For analysis, the left ventricle is divided into segments (Fig. 2.4), with a semi-quantitative analysis of regional wall motion abnormalities. For example, 1 = normokinetic, 2 = hypokinetic, 3 = akinetic, 4 = dyskinetic.[36] Wall motion scores at rest and peak stress are calculated by adding the scores from all segments, with indices for rest and stress wall motion calculated by dividing the scores by the number of segments analysed. The appearance of new or worsening wall motion abnormalities defines a positive test (Fig. 2.5).

Causes of error

It should be noted that segmental wall motion abnormalities, including some changing with stress, do not always indicate ischaemia and can also occur in other cardiac conditions (Table 2.7). These other co-existent conditions should always be considered when interpreting stress echocardiographic images.

Specific indications for stress echocardiography

Detection of myocardial viability

Stress echocardiography, in particular dobutamine echocardiography, is a valuable method for detecting myocardial viability post myocardial infarction, or the functional recovery of hibernating myocardium post-revascularization. On dobutamine echocardiography, hibernating segments show an increased contractility at low doses, due to contractile reserve (i.e. viable myocardium), with an impaired response at high doses (upon development of ischaemia). This biphasic response has a good prognostic value for the recovery of myocardial function following revascularization.[37,38] A biphasic response in an infarcted area can also be used to predict residual stenosis in the infarct-related artery.[39]

Acknowledgements

M.R.B. is supported by a British Heart Foundation Senior Fellowship.

References

1. Bella G, Myocardial perfusion imaging for detection of silent myocardial ischaemia, *Am J Cardiol* 1988; **61**(S): 22F–6F.

2. Bruce R, Hornsten T, Exercise stress testing in evaluation of patients with ischaemic heart disease, *Prog Cardiovasc Dis* 1969; **11**(371): 371–90.

3. McGuire L, The uses and limits of standard exercise tests, *Arch Intern Med* 1981; **141**: 229–32.

4. Epstein S, Implications of probability analysis on the strategy used for non-invasive detection of coronary artery disease, *Am J Cardiol* 1980; **46**: 491–9.

5. DeTrano R, Gianrossi R, Mulvihill D et al, Exercise-induced ST depression in the diagnosis of multivessel disease: a meta analysis, *J Am Coll Cardiol* 1989; **14**: 1501–8.

6. Gianrossi R, Detrano R, Mulvihill D, Exercise-induced ST depression in the diagnosis of coronary artery disease, *Circulation* 1989; **80**: 87–98.

7. Theroux P, Waters D, Halphen C, Debaisieux J, Mizgala H, Prognostic value of exercise testing soon after myocardial infarction, *N Engl J Med* 1979; **301**: 3–6.

8. Saunamaki K, Andersen J, Clinical significance of the ST-segment response and other early exercise variables in uncomplicated vs. complicated myocardial infarction, *Eur Heart J* 1987; **8**: 603.

9. Weld F, Chu K, Bigger JJ, Rolnitzky L, Risk

stratification with low level exercise testing 2 weeks after myocardial infarction, *Circulation* 1981; **64**: 306.

10. Jennings K, Reid D, Hawkins T, Julian D, Role of exercise testing after myocardial infarction in identifying candidates for coronary artery surgery, *Br Med J* 1984; **288**: 185.

11. Weich H, Strauss H, Pitt B, The extraction of thallium-210 by the myocardium, *Circulation* 1977; **56**: 188–91.

12. Leppo J, Myocardial uptake of thallium and rubidium during alterations in perfusion and oxygenation in isolated rabbit hearts, *J Nucl Med* 1987; **28**: 875–85.

13. Melon P, Beanlands S, DeGrado R, Nguyen N, Petry N, Schwaiger M, Comparison of technetium-99m sestamibi and thallium-201 retention characteristics in canine myocardium, *J Am Coll Cardiol* 1992; **20**: 1277–83.

14. Berman D, Kiat H, Vantrain K, Germano G, Maddahi J, Friedman J, Myocardial imaging with technetium-99m-sestamibi — comparative analysis of available imaging protocols, *J Nucl Med* 1994; **35**: 681–8.

15. Weiss A, Berman D, Lew A et al, Transient ischaemic dilatation of the left ventricle on stress thallium-201 scintigraphy: a marker of severe and extensive coronary artery disease, *J Am Coll Cardiol* 1987; **9**: 752–9.

16. Weiss A, Maddahi J, Lew AS et al, Reverse redistribution of thallium-201: a sign of nontransmural myocardial infarction with patency of the infarct-related coronary artery, *J Am Coll Cardiol* 1986; **7**: 61–7.

17. Hirzel H, Senn M, Nuesch K et al, Thallium-201 scintigraphy in complete left bundle branch block, *Am J Cardiol* 1984; **53**: 764–9.

18. O'Keefe J, Bateman T, Barnhart C, Adenosine thallium-201 is superior to exercise thallium-201 for detecting coronary artery disease in patients with left bundle branch block, *J Am Coll Cardiol* 1993; **21**: 1332–8.

19. Jazmati B, Sadaniantz A, Emaus S, Heller G, Exercise thallium-201 imaging in complete left bundle branch block and the prevalence of septal perfusion defects, *Am J Cardiol* 1991; **67**: 46–9.

20. Kotler T, Diamond G, Exercise thallium-201 scintigraphy in the diagnosis and prognosis of coronary artery disease, *Arch Intern Med* 1990; **113**: 684–702.

21. Leppo J, Dipyridamole-thallium imaging: the lazy man's stress test, *J Nucl Med* 1989; **30**: 281–7.

22. Verani M, Adenosine stress imaging, *Cor Art Dis* 1993; **3**: 1145–51.

23. Morise A, Detrano R, Bobbio M, Diamond G, Development and validation of a logistic regression-derived algorithm for estimating the incremental probability of coronary artery disease before and after exercise testing, *J Am Coll Cardiol* 1992; **20**: 1187–96.

24. Abouantoun A, Ahnve S, Savvides M, Witztum K, Jensen D, Froelicher V, Can areas of myocardial ischaemia be localised by the exercise electrocardiogram? A correlative study with thallium-201 scintigraphy, *Am J Heart* 1984; **108**: 933–41.

25. Brown K, Prognostic value of thallium-201 myocardial perfusion imaging. A diagnostic tool comes of age, *Circulation* 1991; **83**: 363–81.

26. Steinberg E, Koss J, Lee M, Grunwald A, Bodenheimer M, Prognostic significance from 10 year follow-up of a qualitatively normal planar exercise thallium test in suspected

coronary artery disease, *Am J Cardiol* 1993; 71: 1270–3.

27. Machecourt J, Longere P, Fagret D et al, Prognostic value of thallium-201 single photon emission computed tomographic myocardial perfusion imaging according to extent of myocardial defect, *J Am Coll Cardiol* 1994; **23**: 1096–106.

28. Eitzman D, Al-Aouar Z, Kanter H et al, Clinical outcome of patients with advanced coronary artery disease after viability studies with positron emission tomography, *J Am Coll Cardiol* 1992; **20**: 559–65.

29. DiCarli M, Davidson M, Little R et al, Value of metabolic imaging with positron emission tomography for evaluating prognosis in patients with coronary artery disease and left ventricular dysfunction, *Am J Cardiol* 1994; 744: 527–33.

30. Tamaki M, Yonekura Y, Yamashita K et al, Positron emission tomography using fluorine-18-deoxyglucose in evaluation of coronary artery bypass grafting, *Am J Cardiol* 1989; **64**: 860–5.

31. Martin T, Seaworth J, Johns J, Comparison of exercise electrocardiography and dobutamine echocardiography, *Clin Cardiol* 1992; **15**: 641–6.

32. Rallidis L, Cokkinos P, Tousoulis D, Nihoyannopoulos P, Comparison of dobutamine and treadmill exercise echocardiography in inducing ischaemia in patients with coronary artery disease, *J Am Coll Cardiol* 1997; **30**: 1660–8.

33. Cohen J, Ottenweller J, George A, Duvvuvi S, Comparison of dobutamine and exercise echocardiography, *Am J Cardiol* 1993; **72**: 1226–33.

34. Marcovitz P, Bachs D, Mathias W, Shayna V, Armstrong W, Paradoxic hypotension during dobutamine stress echocardiography: clinical and diagnostic implications, *J Am Coll Cardiol* 1993; **21**: 1080–6.

35. Poldermans D, Fioretti P, Boersma E et al, Safety of dobutamine–atropine stress echocardiography in patients with suspected or proven coronary artery disease, *Am J Cardiol* 1994; **73**: 456–9.

36. Sawada S, Segar D, Ryan T et al, Echocardiographic detection of coronary artery disease during dobutamine infusion, *Circulation* 1991; **83**: 1605–14.

37. Afridi I, Kleinman N, Raizner A, Zoghbi W, Dobutamine infusion in myocardial hibernation. Optimal dose and accuracy in predicting recovery of ventricular function after coronary angioplasty, *Circulation* 1995; **91**: 661–70.

38. La Canna G, Alfieri O, Giullini R, Gargano M, Ferrari R, Visioli O, Echocardiography during infusion of dobutamine for identification of reversible dysfunction in patients with coronary artery disease, *J Am Coll Cardiol* 1994; **23**: 617–23.

39. Smart S, Knickelbine T, Stoiber T, Carlos M, Wynsen J, Sagar K, Safety and accuracy of dobutamine–atropine stress echocardiography for the detection of residual stenosis of the infarct-related artery and multi-vessel disease during the first week after myocardial infarction, *Circulation* 1997; **95**: 1394–401.

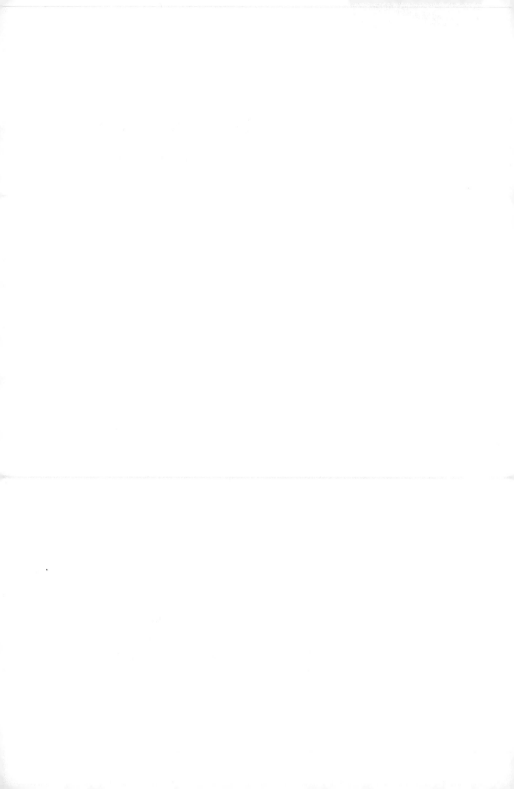

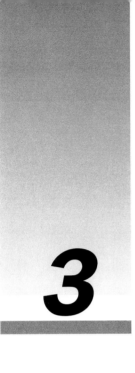

Management of risk factors (i.e. secondary prevention)

Paul D Flynn

3

Introduction

The aim of treating patients is to reduce both the morbidity and the mortality associated with their illness. In the case of angina this means decreasing the severity and frequency of chest pain and reducing the risk of myocardial infarction and cardiac death. It is now well established that patients with overt coronary artery disease are between five and seven times more likely to suffer from myocardial infarction or cardiac death than asymptomatic individuals.[1] In absolute terms the annual rate of infarction has been about 6% in the control groups of the secondary prevention trials, compared with 1–2% in the corresponding groups of the primary prevention trials. Given the prevalence of coronary artery disease, measures that reduce this excess risk could prevent a large number of myocardial infarctions each year.

The concept has already been introduced that there are a number of genetic and environmental factors, such as cigarette smoking, hyperlipidaemia and hypertension, associated with an increased risk of developing coronary artery disease (Fig. 3.1). Not all these risk factors are modifiable,

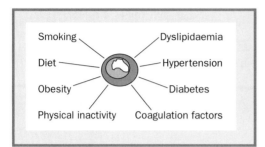

Figure 3.1
The major modifiable coronary risk factors. The major established risk factors discussed in this chapter are shown converging on a diseased coronary artery. 'Lifestyle' factors are shown on the left and other factors on the right, but in reality there are many interactions between these different risk factors. Unmodifiable risk factors and emerging risk factors are not shown.

and it does not necessarily follow that because some condition is associated with the development of coronary disease, altering that factor will reduce the progression or complication rate of disease once it is present. This chapter will review for each modifiable risk factor whether intervention is beneficial.

Changes in lifestyle

Of the modifiable coronary risk factors, a number involve personal habits of smoking, diet, exercise and alcohol consumption. In many ways these represent an ideal target for intervention: they involve no direct cost, are less likely to produce side-effects than pharmacological treatments, and benefit may well not be restricted to a reduction in coronary events. However, changes in lifestyle are notoriously difficult to introduce, or at least maintain, and do not easily lend themselves to placebo-controlled studies.

Clearly, they can never be double-blind, and it can be difficult to quantify changes in diet and exercise. Additionally, information about possible risk factors is rapidly disseminated and may produce changes in the control arm of any study. As most studies are analysed on an intention-to-treat basis, a lack of beneficial effect may tell us more about the difficulty of introducing effective change than about the potential efficacy of that change. We should avoid ignoring that which is difficult to measure, but we also need to obtain as clear evidence as we can before investing, or asking our patients to invest, the time and energy needed to change lifestyle.

Smoking

There is now no doubt that smoking, particularly cigarette smoking, is associated with an increased risk of myocardial infarction and premature cardiac death, as well as chronic pulmonary disease and a variety of cancers, most notably lung cancer. A large number of studies have shown an increased risk of vascular death in current smokers, the average relative risk being 1.7.[2] The risk increases with the number of cigarettes smoked, is present with a consumption as low as 1–5 cigarettes a day, and is not much altered by smoking a low-tar brand. The median life-expectancy for smokers is 72 years; for lifelong non-smokers it is 79.5, representing an additional 7.5 years of life.[3] The greatest benefit of cessation is seen in those who stop smoking before the age of 35, but even stopping between 65 and 75 decreases mortality rates. Half of all smokers will die of their habit and at least half of these deaths will be cardiovascular. Following cessation there is a rapid initial decline in the risk of coronary events, although it may take 10–20 years for the risk to equal that of those who have never smoked.[4] Even in patients with established coronary artery disease there is a reduction in mortality within a year of cessation.[2] In the Coronary Artery Surgery Study, stopping smoking at the time of diagnosis reduced the 5-year mortality rate by a third from 22% to 15%.[5] It is worth noting that in this study 57% of smokers continued even after angiography showed the presence of coronary disease.

Despite the widespread recognition of the risks of continuing to smoke, cessation remains difficult. More than 90% of those who give up resume the habit within 1 year.[6] In an effort to overcome this, various medications delivering nicotine have been developed to help with the symptoms of withdrawal. Of these, the most popular have been chewing gum and transdermal preparations, though a nicotine inhaler has recently been launched. Trials of nicotine medications have generally shown a 2-4-fold increase in the numbers who successfully stop smoking, but only when they are administered as part of a structured programme with follow-up and counselling. It is sad that when even the tobacco companies recognize that nicotine is an addictive substance, no help is offered to those who wish to stop smoking (at least in the UK), in direct contradistinction to those addicted to alcohol or other drugs. While such formal support is not available, it is at least worth exploring every avenue in helping any patient with coronary disease to give up smoking.

Diet

Epidemiological studies have shown a clear association between diets rich in fat, especially saturated fat, and high serum cholesterol levels and the risk of coronary disease. The American Heart Association (AHA) Step II diet recommends restricting the fat content to less than 30% of the total calories, the saturated fat to less than 7% of total calories, and the daily cholesterol intake to less than 200 mg/day. Such diets are effective in reducing total and LDL cholesterol and triglycerides and increasing HDL cholesterol, and have been shown to reduce progression of coronary disease in angiographic studies. However, trials of low-fat diets have generally proved rather disappointing in the secondary prevention of coronary events, partly because the studies have tended to be relatively small and short term and to exclude those patients likely to comply. In contrast, some other dietary interventions have shown clear evidence of benefit in patients with pre-existing coronary disease. In particular, increasing fish oil consumption in the DART trial decreased mortality by 29% over 2 years following myocardial infarction.[7] Even more strikingly, a trial of the Mediterranean diet rich in fresh fruit and vegetables, fish and olive oil produced a 70% reduction in overall mortality and a 76% reduction in coronary mortality in patients with a previous myocardial infarction.[8] The diet was comparatively rich in alpha-linolenic acid and oleic acid and in natural antioxidants, but did not alter serum lipid levels. In a third study, a low-fat diet supplemented with fruit and vegetables and grain products reduced coronary events by 39% and total mortality by 45% compared with a low-fat diet alone.[9] Therefore, encouraging a diet rich in fish oil, antioxidants and oleic and linolenic acids may be at least as important as restricting the fat

content and forms part of the recommendations for healthy eating in both the AHA[10] and the Second European Task Force[11] guidelines.

Another dietary factor to be considered is alcohol. There is now considerable evidence that moderate consumption of alcohol reduces vascular risk by about a third, and is consequently associated with reduced overall mortality.[12] The form of alcohol (wine, beer or spirits) does not appear to matter, and maximal benefit is achieved with an intake of between 14 and 21 units per week in men and slightly less in women. In advising patients of the beneficial effects of alcohol, the adverse consequences of excess consumption, namely the increased risk of accidents, liver disease, cardiomyopathy, hyperlipidaemia, obesity and hypertension, need also to be borne in mind.

Physical activity

The concept that regular physical exercise may be beneficial in patients with coronary artery disease is as old as the description of the disease itself. Heberden himself advocated chopping wood for 30 min each day as a remedy for angina. Regular exercise has a number of physiological effects which may reduce the risk of coronary events, not least lowering low-density lipoprotein (LDL) cholesterol and triglycerides and increasing high-density lipoprotein (HDL) cholesterol and insulin sensitivity. A number of randomized clinical trials have shown that regular physical exercise can reduce cardiovascular mortality by between 20% and 25% following myocardial infarction.[13] It seems reasonable to assume that a similar benefit would be seen in patients with other evidence of coronary artery disease. Clearly, a detailed assessment of patients with angina, including an exercise test if necessary, is required before an appropriate level of exercise can be recommended. Both the AHA[10] and the European[11] guidelines recommend at least 30 min of moderate-level aerobic exercise four or five times a week in patients who have recovered from a myocardial infarction. Heberden seems to have been vindicated!

Obesity

Increasing physical activity, together with calorie restriction, are often required in the management of obesity in secondary prevention. A number of studies have shown that obesity, particularly central obesity, is associated with an increased risk of coronary events, and predicts outcome following revascularization.[14] While the strength of this association is weakened in multivariate analysis including hypertension, diabetes mellitus and hyperlipidaemia, these factors often result from, or at least are exacerbated by, the presence of obesity. There has been no prospective trial examining the benefit of reducing body weight in patients with coronary disease, but it is generally recommended that such patients who are overweight (either body mass index greater than 25 kg/m² or waist circumference greater than 94 cm in men or 80 cm in women) be given advice on weight reduction.[10,11]

Dyslipidaemia

For many years, evidence has been growing that treatment to reduce total and LDL cholesterol is an effective way of reducing the risk of coronary events, especially in those who already have evidence of coronary disease. Until recently, the treatments for hypercholesterolaemia had a relatively minor effect on blood lipid levels, or a wide range of side-effects, or both. Nonetheless, with the notable exception of clofibrate, these treatments were shown to decrease coronary morbidity and mortality, though without a significant reduction in overall mortality.[15] It was even suggested that the beneficial effect on coronary disease was counterbalanced by an increased risk of cancer and suicide. The advent of the HMG-CoA reductase inhibitors (or statins), which produce substantial reductions in total and HDL cholesterol and are well tolerated, has allowed these fears to be addressed definitively. Recently, three major trials of cholesterol reduction using simvastatin or pravastatin in patients with coronary disease and with total cholesterols

Table 3.1
The major lipid-lowering trials in secondary prevention.

	4S	CARE	LIPID
No. in study	4444	4159	9014
Inclusion criteria			
Clinical	MI or angina	MI	MI or unstable angina
Total cholesterol	5.5–8.0 mM	<6.2 mM (LDL-C 3.0–4.5 mM)	4.0–7.0 mM
Triglycerides	≤2.5 mM	<3.95 mM	≤5.0 mM
Treatment	Simvastatin 10–40 mg	Pravastatin 40 mg	Pravastatin 40 mg
Follow-up	5.4 years	5.0 years	6.1 years
Effect on lipids			
Total cholesterol	↓ 25%	↓ 20%	↓ 18%
LDL-cholesterol	↓ 35%	↓ 28%	↓ 35%
HDL-cholesterol	↑ 8%	↑ 5%	↑ 5%
Triglycerides	↓ 10%	↓ 14%	↓ 11%
Outcome			
Total mortality	↓ 30% ($p = 0.0003$)		↓ 22% ($p < 0.001$)
Coronary death	↓ 42%		↓ 24% ($p < 0.001$)
Major coronary events	↓ 34% ($p < 0.00001$)	↓ 24% ($p = 0.003$)	↓ 24% ($p < 0.001$)

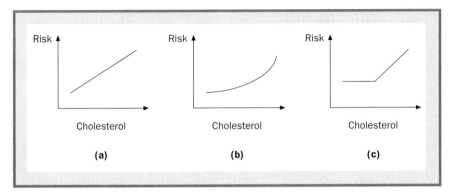

Figure 3.2
Models of the relationship between cholesterol and coronary risk.
Three possible models of the relationship between risk of coronary disease and cholesterol are shown; a
linear model (a), a curvilinear model (b) and a threshold model (c).

ranging from 4.0 to 8.0 mM have been completed (Table 3.1).[16–18] These trials have confirmed that reducing cholesterol lowers the incidence of myocardial infarction and coronary death, and the need for revascularization procedures. The Scandinavian Simvastatin Survival Study [4S] and the Long-term Intervention with Pravastatin in Ischaemic Disease (LIPID) study both showed a significant reduction in overall mortality, with no increase in the risk of death from cancer, suicide or other cause in the treated group.[16,18] As an additional benefit, the trials all showed a significant reduction in the risk of stroke. It is now clear that cholesterol reduction with the statins is safe and effective in the management of patients with coronary artery disease.

Nonetheless, several questions remain. Chief among these are whether all patients with coronary artery disease should be treated with a statin and by how much the LDL cholesterol should be reduced. Current guidance on these issues is largely derived from subgroup analysis of the lipid-lowering trials, and so may have to be reviewed as further evidence becomes available. Central to these questions is the nature of the relationship between total or LDL cholesterol and the risk of coronary events.[19] The earlier studies provide clear evidence that this relationship is logarithmic for total cholesterols greater than 4.0 mM.[15] Does the same model hold for the lower values seen following treatment in the recent trials, or is a threshold model more applicable (Fig. 3.2)?

Analysis of the 4S study patients divided into quintiles showed that both the absolute level and the change in LDL cholesterol with treatment correlated with risk of coronary events; pairwise analysis was unable to determine which of the two related measures was the more important.[19] The risk of coronary events decreased with treatment LDL cholesterol levels down to 2.2 mM, with no evidence of a threshold below which further benefit was not seen, in accord with earlier evidence.[15] However, the incremental benefit became progressively less as the LDL reduction increased. The Cholesterol and Recurrent Events (CARE) study showed a significant reduction in coronary events in all patients with a baseline LDL cholesterol level greater than 3.2 mM, which represents about 80% of all coronary disease patients in North America.[17] However, patients with a baseline LDL cholesterol less than 3.2 mM experienced no reduction in coronary events with treatment, but the numbers were relatively small and the confidence intervals correspondingly wide.[17] Similarly, while LDL cholesterol (on treatment) was significantly correlated with coronary risk in the CARE study, the relationship was not linear, with no fall in relative risk at LDL cholesterol values less than 3.2 mM.[19] However, as the relationship between LDL cholesterol and risk was deduced by examining relative risk in deciles of the study population, the data probably do not allow distinction between a curvilinear and a threshold model. The LIPID study found no evidence of significant heterogeneity of effect in the various prespecified subgroups, including stratification by lipid levels.[18] On balance, most of the evidence suggests that the relationship between LDL cholesterol and coronary risk is a curvilinear one, even down to the very low LDL cholesterol levels seen in the most recent trials.

In conclusion, current evidence suggests that there are very few patients with coronary artery disease who would not benefit from a statin. The ideal aim of treatment is to reduce the LDL cholesterol as far as possible. This concept has recently been supported by the Atorvastatin Versus Revascularisation Treatments (AVERT) study, which was reported at the 1998 71st AHA Scientific Sessions. In this study, patients with moderate angina were randomized to angioplasty plus normal treatment or high-dose atorvastatin. Treatment with atorvastatin produced a significant reduction in a combined endpoint of major coronary events or further revascularization, even though 70% of the revascularization arm also received lipid-lowering therapy. The mean LDL cholesterol achieved with high-dose atorvastatin was 2.0 mM. Several other studies (e.g. SEARCH and TNT) are underway to further test the hypothesis that greater LDL reduction reduces coronary risk more. The European guidelines recommend that the LDL cholesterol be reduced below 3.0 mM,[11] while the AHA guidelines suggest a target of 2.6 mM,[10] but these did not take account of the data from the AVERT trial and may need to be amended in the light of this and ongoing studies.

Debate has also developed over whether the benefit seen in the statin trials has been entirely due to their effect on LDL cholesterol. The West of Scotland Coronary Prevention (WOSCOPS) trial was predominantly a trial of pravastatin in primary prevention, but did include a number of patients with angina. In a post-hoc analysis of a subgroup of the WOSCOPS study, treated subjects had a lower rate of coronary events than controls with very similar LDL cholesterol levels.[19] The observed risk in the controls was accurately predicted by the Framingham risk equation, but was overestimated in the treatment group. This has led to suggestions that statins may have a beneficial effect in coronary disease over and above their effect on lipids, and it has been shown that they do have pleiotropic effects on atherogenic processes 'in vitro'. Nonetheless, even in the recent statin trials the overall reduction in risk is much as would be predicted from the change in LDL cholesterol,[15] which suggests that most of the benefit of the statins is due to their lipid-lowering properties.

So far I have concentrated entirely on LDL cholesterol, but in fact the commonest dyslipidaemia in patients with coronary disease comprises low HDL cholesterol, high triglycerides and a predominance of small dense LDL particles; the so-called atherogenic lipid phenotype. In the treatment groups of 4S and WOSCOPS, baseline HDL cholesterol and triglycerides were significant, though not independent, predictors of coronary event rate. Change in HDL cholesterol correlated with risk in 4S, but not in CARE or WOSCOPS, and change in triglyceride correlated with risk in CARE but not 4S or WOSCOPS.[19] It is worth noting that high triglycerides were an exclusion criterion in these studies (Table 3.1). Although the statins do have beneficial effects on levels of HDL cholesterol and triglycerides, the magnitude of these changes is small. There is little evidence on the effect of increasing HDL cholesterol or lowering triglycerides in patients with coronary disease. The Bezafibrate Coronary Atherosclerosis Intervention Trial (BECAIT) was a randomized trial of the effect of bezafibrate on angiographic progression of coronary artery disease in men following a myocardial infarction.[20] Treatment significantly retarded progression of disease, and even significantly reduced the number of coronary events (though the numbers involved were very small), despite reducing LDL cholesterol by only 2%. However, bezafibrate did decrease triglycerides by 31% and increase HDL cholesterol by 9%. In the Helsinki Heart Study, gemfibrozil reduced coronary events by 34% over 5 years in primary prevention.[21] Again, the reduction in LDL cholesterol was modest at 8%, but triglycerides were reduced by 35% and HDL cholesterol increased by 9%. Preliminary results from the Bezafibrate Infarction Prevention (BIP) study were announced at the 1998 European Society of Cardiology meeting. Bezafibrate produced a moderate, but non-significant, reduction in acute coronary events in patients with a previous history of myocardial infarction or angina pectoris. However, in the subgroup with triglycerides between 2.2 and 3.4 mM, the 40% reduction in the combined endpoint was significant. It is perhaps not surprising that bezafibrate, with its minimal reduction in LDL cholesterol, is not effective in secondary prevention in pure hypercholesterolaemia, but these studies do suggest that focusing exclusively on LDL cholesterol may not always be appropriate. In considering the treatment of patients with coronary disease and the atherogenic lipoprotein phenotype it is still clear that the first aim of treatment should be to reduce LDL cholesterol, but treatment to increase HDL cholesterol and reduce triglycerides where these are also deranged may confer additional benefit, as is recommended in the AHA guidelines.[10]

Hypertension

Epidemiological studies have shown a clear correlation between blood pressure and the risk of cardiovascular and cerebrovascular disease, with a difference in diastolic blood pressure of 5–6 mmHg being associated with a 20–25% difference in the prevalence of coronary disease and a 35–40% difference in the prevalence of stroke.[22] Additionally, hypertension is one of the commonest causes of chronic renal failure, which is itself associated with the development of obliterative vascular disease. Meta-analysis of the earlier trials of reducing blood pressure (predominantly using beta-blockers or diuretics) showed that the mean reduction of diastolic blood pressure of 5–6 mmHg reduced stroke by 42% even within the 2–3-year duration of the trials, which is close to the predicted value.[22,23] Although there was also a significant reduction in coronary events, the 14% reduction was rather less than would have been expected from the observational studies. The reason for this shortfall remains unclear. Overall vascular mortality was reduced by 21%, with no significant difference in non-vascular mortality. When the more recent trials in the elderly were included, stroke was reduced by 38% and coronary disease morbidity and mortality by 16%.[24] Given the high level of absolute risk of coronary events in patients with pre-existing coronary disease, even this relatively modest reduction in relative risk may be worthwhile. Additionally, patients with coronary disease are at higher risk of stroke, and lowering blood pressure gives clear and substantial benefit in the prevention of cerebrovascular events.

The target for treatment of hypertension has been addressed in the recent Hypertension Optimal Treatment (HOT) study.[25] Hypertensive patients were randomized to have their diastolic blood pressure (DBP) reduced to ≤90 mmHg, ≤85 mmHg or ≤80 mmHg, using treatment regimens based on the long-acting calcium channel blocker felodipine and including an angiotensin-converting enzyme (ACE) inhibitor, beta-blocker or diuretic as required. While the coronary event rates were lower than predicted, hinting at the efficacy of the intensive treatment in this trial, the differences between the three groups were small and only the trend for the rate of myocardial infarction to be lower at a lower target blood pressure achieved borderline significance. It was concluded that most of the benefit of lowering blood pressure was achieved when the DBP was reduced to 90 mmHg and the systolic to 140 mmHg.

The HOT study included a substantial number of patients with a previous history of myocardial infarction or other evidence of coronary disease. As for the complete study group, the trend for a reduction in coronary events with more intensive treatment was not significant, but the reduction in stroke was significant with a 43% lower incidence in the group with a target DBP of ≤80 mmHg compared with the group with a target DBP of ≤90 mmHg.[25]

In treating hypertension, advice should be given about dietary salt restriction, alcohol consumption and weight reduction where appropriate. A number of classes of antihypertensive drugs are available if pharmacological intervention is also required, and many of the trials of lowering blood pressure have used combinations of these agents. Not surprisingly, there is more evidence of the safety and efficacy of the older agents, such as beta-blockers and thiazides. In particular, beta-blockers have been associated with a 25% reduction in the recurrence of coronary events and vascular mortality following myocardial infarction.[26] The benefit is seen even in those with a DBP less than 70 mmHg, suggesting that beta-blockers may exert some specific cardioprotective effect in this situation. Patients with angina and a preceding history of myocardial infarction should therefore be treated with a beta-blocker regardless of their blood pressure, if there are no contraindications. As the beta-blockers also have anti-anginal properties, they represent a logical choice of antihypertensive in patients with angina even in the absence of previous infarction.

Evidence is also growing of the efficacy of the newer agents. A number of trials have shown that the ACE inhibitors reduce mortality in patients with impaired left ventricular function following myocardial infarction.[27] Where no direct measurement of left ventricular function is possible, it has been suggested that ACE inhibitors should be given to survivors of myocardial infarction when there is clinical evidence of failure, when the infarction is a recurrent event or when there has been full-thickness infarction of the anterior wall.[10,27] Treatment with the ACE inhibitors produces greatest benefit in patients with continuing angina, and is associated, in at least some of the trials, with a reduction in acute coronary events. Trials of ACE inhibitors in angina are underway. An overview of trials of the calcium channel blockers found no evidence of reduced coronary morbidity or mortality despite their symptomatic benefit.[28] However, this result may have been affected by the adverse effects of the short-acting agents, and recent trials with the longer-acting calcium channel blockers have been more encouraging.[25]

In conclusion, both the AHA[10] and the European[11] guidelines recommend reducing blood pressure to less than 140/90 mmHg in secondary prevention. When there is a history of myocardial infarction, treatment should include a beta-blocker; if there is also left ventricular dysfunction, an ACE inhibitor

should be given. In the absence of prior infarction, beta-blockers will help control both blood pressure and symptoms of angina and are of proven benefit, but long-acting calcium channel blockers and other agents may also be helpful.

Diabetes

Diabetes is well recognized as a risk factor for coronary disease. Indeed, much of the excess mortality seen in diabetic patients is accounted for by their three-fold increased risk of cardiovascular disease. Furthermore, the prognosis for patients with coronary disease is worse in diabetics. This increased risk is independent of other risk factors; when patients are stratified for the presence or severity of hypertension, hypercholesterolaemia or cigarette consumption, coronary disease is still more common in diabetics.[29] However, while intensive control of blood sugar levels clearly reduces the incidence of the microvascular complications of diabetes (specifically retinopathy, neuropathy and nephropathy) in both type 1 and type 2 diabetes, the effect on macrovascular disease is equivocal.[30,31] While intensive control in the Diabetes Control and Complications Trial (DCCT) did significantly reduce the frequency of hypercholesterolaemia in type 1 diabetics compared with conventional treatment, the reduction in combined cardiovascular and peripheral vascular endpoint just failed to reach significance.[30] However, the study was conducted in subjects in their 20s and early 30s with a low coronary event rate, raising questions about its power to detect a difference between the two groups. The coronary event rate was much higher in the type 2 diabetics studied in the United Kingdom Prospective Diabetes Study (UKPDS) but again intensive treatment failed to reduce the rate of macrovascular complications.[31] A battery of vascular endpoints were studied, of which only the reduction in non-fatal myocardial infarction reached borderline significance. No trial has specifically addressed the issue of intensive blood glucose control in patients with existing coronary disease. However, it seems that while such treatment is beneficial in reducing microvascular complications, it may have little impact on the macrovascular disease that contributes so much to diabetic mortality, especially given the difficulty of reproducing the intensive conditions of the trials in normal clinical practice.

So what should be done about the burden of coronary disease in diabetics? Diabetics have an increased incidence of hypertension and, for a given systolic blood pressure, are at higher risk of coronary disease than non-diabetics. The HOT Study showed a greater and more significant reduction in the rate of major coronary events with more aggressive blood pressure lowering in the subjects with diabetes compared with those with normal blood sugars.[26] The risk of myocardial infarction was halved in the group with a target DBP of ≤80 mmHg compared with the group with a target DBP of ≤90 mmHg but the difference just failed to achieve significance. Tight control of blood pressure in the UKPDS also significantly reduced the risk of stroke (as well as microvascular disease and overall diabetes-related morbidity and mortality), but produced a smaller and non-significant reduction in myocardial infarction.[32] It may be relevant that the target DBP was 80 mmHg in the HOT Study and 85 mmHg in the UKPDS. It is also worth noting that treatment with either an ACE inhibitor or beta-blocker in the UKPDS retarded progression of microalbuminuria, itself a predictor of coronary risk.[32] So blood pressure reduction seems particularly beneficial in diabetics, and should aim to reduce the DBP well below 90 mmHg to achieve maximal reduction of coronary risk.

As for hypertension, diabetics are at higher risk for coronary disease at any level of total cholesterol. Trials are now underway to investigate the effect of cholesterol reduction in diabetics in both primary and secondary prevention. Subgroup analysis of the 4S and CARE Studies has shown that treatment with an HMG-CoA reductase inhibitor significantly reduced the risk of major coronary events in diabetics with a previous history of myocardial infarction at least as much as in the overall study population.[33] This result is interesting, as the treatment used in these two studies principally lowered total and LDL cholesterol, with only minor changes in triglycerides and HDL cholesterol. While LDL cholesterol is an independent risk factor in diabetics, elevated LDL cholesterol is not the main feature of diabetic dyslipidaemia, which is in fact characterized by increased levels of triglycerides and reduced levels of HDL cholesterol. Some of the trials of lipid modulation in diabetics are testing the hypothesis that increasing HDL cholesterol and reducing triglycerides will further reduce the high level of coronary disease in this population.

In summary, careful monitoring and control of blood sugar is warranted in diabetics with coronary disease to reduce microvascular complications but may not much affect the risk of macrovascular disease. Evidence is emerging that aggressive treatment of hypertension and dyslipidaemia is required to reduce the risk of further coronary disease in this population.

Antiplatelet treatment

The history of the use of antiplatelet agents in the prevention of myocardial infarction differs from that of other risk factors in that it results

more from studies of pathogenesis than of epidemiology. Even today, when some procoagulant factors, such as fibrinogen, have been shown to be associated with vascular disease, there is no marker of platelet activity to allow stratification of risk. This is probably because the stimulus to platelet adhesion and aggregation in vascular occlusion results more from a disruption of the normal anticoagulant properties of the endothelium than from a generalized disturbance of platelet function. Nonetheless, reducing platelet aggregation has proved effective in preventing the complications of vascular disease. The Antiplatelet Trialists' Collaboration reviewed all the trials of antiplatelet agents completed by 1990.[34] In patients with a previous history of myocardial infarction, the risk of the combined endpoint of myocardial infarction, stroke or vascular death was reduced by 25%, of non-fatal myocardial infarction by 31%, of non-fatal stroke by 39%, and of overall mortality by 12%. Changes of similar magnitude were seen in the group considered at high risk because of a history of angina (stable or unstable), revascularization, peripheral arterial disease, or renal disease or diabetes, although the absolute risks were lower. It was estimated that treating 1000 such patients for 2 years with aspirin would prevent 10 deaths and 20 non-fatal vascular events. Only about 600 patients with stable angina were included, but including the more recent Swedish Angina Pectoris Aspirin Trial and the US Physicians' Health Study increased this number to 3000, with a highly significant 33% reduction in vascular events.[34] An aspirin dose of 75 mg/day, which causes almost complete inhibition of platelet cyclo-oxygenase, seemed sufficient to produce the full clinical benefit, except where more rapid inhibition was required.

At the time of the Antiplatelet Trialists' Collaboration, no other antiplatelet agent offered a clear advantage over aspirin. Newer agents include clopidrogel, which inhibits ADP-mediated activation of the platelet glycoprotein IIa/IIIb receptor. In the Clopidrogel versus Aspirin in Patients at Risk of Ischaemic Events (CAPRIE) study, clopidrogel reduced the combined risk of stroke, myocardial infarction or vascular death by 8.7% more than aspirin.[35] If 1000 patients were treated for 2 years with clopidrogel, 10 further events would be prevented. However, while the overall reduction in risk was significant, in the group with a history of myocardial infarction (about 6000 patients) there was no evidence of benefit, compared with a highly significant 23.8% benefit in patients with peripheral arterial disease. Clopidrogel has not been studied in patients with angina (either stable or unstable), but unless it has a greater benefit in this group than the overall effect seen in CAPRIE it would only prevent at most four further events in 1000 patients over 2 years compared with aspirin.

As hypertension particularly increases the risk of haemorrhagic stroke, there has been some concern about the use of aspirin in hypertensives. In the HOT study, aspirin significantly reduced the risk of cardiovascular events by 15% and myocardial infarction by 36%, with no effect on the incidence of stroke or vascular death, in hypertensive subjects.[25] There was no increase in the frequency of fatal bleeds, but both major and minor non-fatal bleeds were significantly increased with a relative risk of 1.8. Overall, there were 53 fewer cardiovascular events in the aspirin group, with 59 more major and 69 more minor bleeds, so that the use of aspirin in hypertensive subjects seems finely balanced. Only 7.5% of the HOT study participants had evidence of coronary disease, and it is possible that aspirin would produce greater benefit in such patients. Conversely, blood pressure was well controlled in this study and the risk of aspirin may be greater where this is not the case. It might therefore be sensible to control blood pressure before instituting aspirin in patients with angina and hypertension.

In summary, there is very clear evidence that aspirin prevents vascular events in patients with angina, whether or not they have a prior history of myocardial infarction, and it should be given to all such patients, though with some caution in those who have co-existent hypertension. No other antiplatelet agent has yet been shown to be superior to aspirin in this group of patients.

Hormone replacement therapy

It is well known that coronary disease is relatively uncommon in premenopausal women, but that risk increases following the menopause and is probably related to oestrogen deficiency. Oestrogen replacement therapy decreases this risk by between 35% and 50%, related in part to improvements in fibrinolytic and lipid parameters and reduced lipid oxidation.[36] However, unopposed oestrogen cannot be given to most post-menopausal females because of the increased risk of uterine cancer. Adding progesterone removes this risk, but also attenuates some of the beneficial effects of oestrogen. Nonetheless, several observational studies have suggested that combined oestrogen–progesterone hormone replacement therapy (HRT) also reduces coronary risk following the menopause. However, the first randomized trial of combined HRT, the Heart and Estrogen/progestin Replacement Study (HERS) was recently completed and showed no effect on the combined endpoint of non-fatal myocardial infarction or coronary death, or any other cardiovascular outcome, in postmenopausal women with coronary disease.[37] Serum lipids were significantly altered; LDL cholesterol was reduced by 14% and HDL cholesterol increased by 8%,

although triglycerides were increased by 10%. There was an increased risk of venous thromboembolism, with 4.1 excess events per 1000 patient years. Clearly, a randomized trial avoids many of the biases inherent in observational studies, but it may be premature to dismiss HRT. While the trial showed a slight overall risk in the first year of treatment, there was a trend towards benefit later and it may be that the trial duration of 4 years was too short to detect benefit. Additionally, the choice of regimen (conjugated equine oestrogens and medroxyprogesterone acetate) may not have been optimal, and as this was a trial of secondary prevention the average age of the participants was nearly 67 years. The discrepancy between this study and the observational data may be resolved by the ongoing WELL-HART and Women's Health Initiative Randomized Trials which are due to report in 2000 and 2005 respectively. For the time being, it is difficult to recommend combined HRT in isolation for secondary prevention of coronary disease in women, although it still has a role in relieving menopausal symptoms and in preventing osteoporosis.

Emerging risk factors
Homocysteine

It has been known for many years that patients with homocystinuria are at increased risk of vascular disease, particularly arterial and venous thromboses. Such patients have extremely high plasma homocysteine concentrations due to genetic deficiency in cystathionine β-synthase, which is a key enzyme in the trans-sulphuration pathway for the conversion of homocysteine to cysteine. In recent years it has become clear that more modest hyperhomocystinaemia is also an independent risk factor for coronary, cerebral and peripheral vascular disease.[38] The odds ratio for a 5 μM increase in plasma homocysteine for coronary disease is 1.6 in men and 1.8 in women, broadly equivalent to an increase in total cholesterol of 0.5 mM. Plasma homocysteine levels are strongly and inversely related to plasma folate levels, and several studies have shown reductions in homocysteine following administration of folic acid, even in patients with normal folate status.[38] Folic acid supplementation of as little as 400 μg/day can reduce plasma homocysteine by up to 6 μM. Even the consumption of two or three more helpings each day of fresh fruit or vegetables would increase folic acid absorption by 50 μg/day, and reduce homocysteine by 2 μM, and should therefore form part of the dietary advice given to patients with angina. Trials are now underway to determine whether folic acid supplementation does reduce vascular risk, and these should be completed before folic acid enrichment of flour and cereals is considered.

Lipid peroxidation

It is also becoming increasingly clear that oxidized LDL cholesterol is more atherogenic than LDL cholesterol itself. Cellular cholesterol uptake by the LDL receptor is subject to negative feedback regulation and is downregulated as intracellular cholesterol increases. However, uptake of oxidized LDL cholesterol by the scavenger receptors is not subject to similar regulation, and it is this pathway that is responsible for the formation of the lipid-laden foam cells that are a characteristic cellular component of the atherosclerotic plaque. Additionally, oxidized LDL cholesterol may increase adhesion molecule expression, monocyte recruitment and vascular smooth muscle cell apoptosis. A number of observational studies have shown an inverse relationship between the consumption of antioxidants (particularly vitamin E or alpha-tocopherol) and the risk of cardiovascular disease.[39] In the Cambridge Heart Antioxidant Study (CHAOS) treatment with alpha-tocopherol (400–800 IU/day) decreased the risk of coronary death or non-fatal myocardial infarction by 47% and the risk of non-fatal myocardial infarction alone by 77% over 17 months in patients with angiographically proven coronary artery disease.[40] However, there were non-significant increases of 18% and 25% in cardiovascular and total mortality. Other studies in patients with previous myocardial infarction or angina pectoris have also found non-significant increases in fatal coronary events with alpha-tocopherol, but did not find any reduction in coronary disease, although these trials used a lower dose than in CHAOS.[41,42] While these discrepancies are explored in further trials, it is probably sensible to restrict advice to patients with angina to increase their antioxidant intake through fresh fruit and vegetables.

Plant sterols

The enrichment of margarines with plant sterols represents a new approach to the reduction of cholesterol on a population basis. Plant sterols inhibit intestinal absorption of cholesterol; normal consumption is between 200 and 400 mg per day. By supplementing margarines it is possible to increase daily consumption to about 3 g/day, and this in turn produces a 6–8% decrease in total cholesterol and a 11–13% reduction in LDL cholesterol compared with a normal polyunsaturated spread.[43] There was no adverse effect on HDL cholesterol. There are some theoretical concerns; some of the plant sterols, such as sitosterol, are themselves absorbed and the rare condition of hereditary sitosterolaemia is characterized by high serum sitosterol concentrations and premature coronary artery disease. To circumvent this problem, at least one of the available agents uses a modified plant sterol, sitostanol, which is not itself absorbed. This approach could

significantly reduce coronary risk, but there is as yet no evidence that these new compounds affect clinical outcome.

Discussion

In summary, there is clear evidence that the natural history of coronary artery disease can be modified by interventions targeted at the known risk factors. To what extent have these findings been translated into clinical practice? The European Action on Secondary Prevention through Intervention to Reduce Events (EUROASPIRE) study suggests that there is considerable scope for improvement.[44] Among patients with various clinical manifestations of coronary artery disease, 19% continued to smoke cigarettes and 25% were overweight with a BMI greater than 30 kg/m^2. Only 32% were receiving lipid-lowering drugs, and of those half still had a total cholesterol greater than 5.5 mM. Only 54% were receiving beta-blockers and 30% ACE inhibitors (58% and 38% respectively in those with a prior history of myocardial infarction). Fifty-three per cent had high blood pressure which was not always treated, and even when it was, half the patients still had a systolic blood pressure greater than 140 mmHg, and in a fifth the systolic blood pressure was greater than 160 mmHg. Perhaps the one redeeming feature was that 81% of the patients were receiving antiplatelet therapy. What is even more depressing is that this study was carried out in a number of European centres in 1995–96, when much of the evidence discussed in this chapter was already published.

There are perhaps a number of reasons why the clear results of the clinical trials have not been more widely carried through to clinical practice. There will always be some delay in disseminating the results of trials; there is a natural and correct caution of physicians to avoid doing their patients harm; and many of these studies have been subjected to controversial analysis. There are practical difficulties too: certainly in the UK, the time available for a full risk factor assessment and discussion of the interventions required is limited. Finally, there are obviously considerable cost implications of treating the large number of patients with coronary disease with a cocktail of drugs, all of which have to be given indefinitely and some of which are relatively expensive.

In fact, most economic analyses of the secondary prevention measures described in this chapter find them to be cost-effective. Such analyses are based on the number of events prevented or lives saved by particular treatments. In any trial this absolute risk reduction will depend on both the initial absolute risk and the relative reduction in that risk. Table 3.2 shows a crude analysis of both measures from the major studies discussed in

this chapter. It is worth noting just how many of the interventions have been shown to improve survival in addition to reducing coronary morbidity.

It is also striking that most of the measures produce similar relative risk reductions of 20–30% in overall mortality and major coronary events. However, these similar relative risk reductions do translate into more variable absolute risk reductions, measured as the number of events prevented per 1000 patient years of treatment. These differences in absolute benefit arise mainly from differences in the initial absolute risk of the populations studied. Initial absolute risk tends to be higher in the earlier studies, in accord with the observed decline in coronary mortality and morbidity in many populations over the past 20 years. Even in patients with a previous history of myocardial infarction, the absolute risk of coronary events differs substantially between countries, as illustrated by the relatively low event rate in the placebo arm of the 4S study. Thus it is not possible to use the absolute benefits calculated from the different trials to compare the efficacy of the interventions, except in similar populations. Nonetheless, it is clear that where particularly high-risk patients can be selected, absolute benefit tends to be greater, as seen in the AIRE study.

One point about most of the trials discussed

Table 3.2
Absolute and relative risk reductions in the major trials of secondary prevention.

Risk factor	Study	Treatment	Patients	Absolute risk: placebo	Absolute risk: treatment	Events prevented	Relative risk reduction (%)	Type of event
Smoking	CASS[5]	Cessation	Post-CABG	44.0	30.0	14.0	31.8	Deaths
Diet	DART[7]	Fish oils	MI	64.0	46.5	17.5	27.3	Deaths
	Mediterranean[8]	α-Linolenic acid	MI	33.7	13.2	20.5	61.4	Deaths
				55.5	13.2	42.3	76.2	MCEs
Lipids	4S[16]	Simvastatin	MI or angina	19.1	13.3	5.8	30.4	Deaths
				46.6	32.3	14.3	30.7	MCEs
	CARE[17]	Pravastatin	MI	26.4	20.4	6.0	22.7	MCEs
	LIPID[18]	Pravastatin	MI or unstable angina	23.0	18.1	4.9	21.5	Deaths
				26.0	20.2	5.8	22.3	MCEs
Blood pressure	Meta-analysis[26]	Beta-blockers	MI	61.9	48.9	13.0	21.0	Deaths
	SAVE[27]	Captopril	MI, LVEF <40%	67.5	55.0	12.5	18.5	Deaths
	AIRE[27]	Ramipril	MI, clinical heart failure	77.5	60.0	17.5	22.6	MCEs
				124.0	92.0	32.0	25.8	Deaths
Coagulation	Meta-analysis[34]	Aspirin	MI	104.0	92.0	12.0	11.5	Deaths
				171.0	135.0	36.0	21.0	MCEs
			Other high risk	48.0	41.0	7.0	14.6	Deaths
				92.0	69.0	27.0	29.3	MCEs

The table shows the absolute risk (in terms of number of events per 1000 patient years) with and without treatment in each of the major trials or meta-analyses referred to in this chapter, and the absolute (also per 1000 patient years) and relative risk reductions for each of the interventions. Reductions are shown for overall mortality and for major coronary events (MCEs), the latter being defined as the sum of coronary death and non-fatal myocardial infarction (MI) except for the aspirin meta-analysis, where strokes are also included in the total. Only significant reductions are included. LVEF, left ventricular ejection fraction.

in this chapter is that they have not focused exclusively on patients with stable or unstable angina, with the exception of the AVERT study. However, the relative risk reductions in this study and in the trials of interventions in primary prevention are similar to those seen when there has been a previous major coronary event. As the absolute risk is lower in patients without a history of myocardial infarction, the absolute benefit of intervention will also be lower, but, as the Antiplatelet Trialists' Collaboration illustrates, in patients with uncomplicated angina both these measures are still above the threshold at which intervention is considered worthwhile (taken as an annual risk of a major coronary event greater than 2–3%).

Conclusion

In summary, patients with angina are at sufficiently high risk of coronary morbidity and mortality that attempts to reduce that risk are justifiable. Such patients should be given advice about stopping smoking, dietary modification, regular exercise and weight loss. In addition, they should all receive antiplatelet and lipid-lowering treatment, and the LDL cholesterol should be reduced to less than 3.0 mM at most. All patients with a history of myocardial infarction should receive a beta-blocker, and if there is any evidence of left ventricular dysfunction an ACE inhibitor. Blood pressure should be reduced to less than

140/90 mmHg. Diabetic patients warrant aggressive blood pressure and lipid lowering. More detailed advice and treatment aims can be found in the AHA and European Task Force guidelines.[10,11]

There is still much to be done to translate research studies into clinical practice. Sometimes it appears that more effort goes into discovering new risk factors than in modifying those where intervention has already been shown to be beneficial. Often it seems that a particular risk factor is singled out for attention and the others neglected. Most patients who develop coronary disease do so as the result of an interaction of several risk factors, and it seems likely that they will benefit most from interventions targeted at all the risk factors present. The situation may be analogous to an examination where it is better to attempt all the questions rather than just answering one or two extremely well.

A final point is that it is increasingly clear that much of the risk of developing coronary disease is genetic, and therefore inherited. In patients who present with premature coronary disease, this genetic contribution is likely to be particularly significant. It follows that the relatives of such patients should be screened for the presence of modifiable risk factors, but in the EUROASPIRE study only 21% of coronary disease patients had been advised that their relatives should be so screened. The

European Task Force guidelines[11] suggest that such advice should at least be given to males presenting before the age of 55 years and females before the age of 60 years.

References

1. Rossouw J, Lewis B, Rifkind BM, The value of lowering cholesterol after myocardial infarction, *N Engl J Med* 1990; **323**: 1112–19.

2. McBride PE, The health consequences of smoking, *Med Clin North Am* 1992; **76**: 333–53.

3. Doll R, Peto R, Wheatley K, Gray R, Sutherland I, Mortality in relation to smoking: 40 years' observations on British doctors, *Br Med J* 1994; **309**: 901–11.

4. Samet JM, The health benefits of smoking cessation, *Med Clin North Am* 1992; **76**: 399–414.

5. Vlietstra RE, Kronmal RA, Oberman A et al, Effect of cigarette smoking on survival of patients with angiographically documented coronary artery disease. Report from the CASS registry, *JAMA* 1986; **255**: 1023–7.

6. Henningfield JE, Nicotine medications for smoking cessation, *N Engl J Med* 1995; **333**: 1196–203.

7. Burr ML, Gilbert JF, Holliday RM et al, Effects of changes in fat, fish and fibre intakes on death and myocardial reinfarction: diet and reinfarction trial, *Lancet* 1989; **ii**: 757–61.

8. de Lorgeril M, Renaud S, Mamelle N et al, Mediterranean alpha-linolenic acid-rich diet in secondary prevention of coronary heart disease, *Lancet* 1994; **343**: 1454–9.

9. Singh RB, Rastogi SS, Verma R et al, Randomised trial of cardioprotective diet in patients with recent acute myocardial infarction: results of one year follow up, *Br Med J* 1992; **304**: 1015–19.

10. Smith SC Jr, Blair SN, Criqui MH et al, AHA Medical/Scientific Statement. Consensus Panel Statement. Preventing heart attack and death in patients with coronary disease, *Circulation* 1995; **92**: 2–4.

11. Wood D, De Backer G, Faergeman O, Graham I, Mancia G, Pyörälä K, Prevention of coronary heart disease in clinical practice. Recommendations of the second joint task force of European and other societies on coronary prevention, *Eur Heart J* 1998; **19**: 1434–503.

12. Doll R, One for the heart, *Br Med J* 1997; **315**: 1664–8.

13. Bernadet P, Benefits of physical activity in the prevention of cardiovascular diseases, *J Cardiovasc Pharmacol* 1995; **25**(suppl. 1): S3–8.

14. Prasad US, Walker WS, Sang CT, Campanella C, Cameron EW, Influence of obesity on the early and long-term results of surgery for coronary artery disease, *Eur J Cardiothorac Surg* 1991; **5**: 67–72.

15. Law MR, Wald NJ, Thompson SG et al, The cholesterol papers, *Br Med J* 1994; **308**: 363–79.

16. Pedersen TR, Kjekshus J, Berg K et al, Randomised trial of cholesterol lowering in 4444 patients with coronary heart disease: the Scandinavian Simvastatin Survival Study (4S), *Lancet* 1994; **344**: 1383–9.

17. Sacks FM, Pfeffer MA, Moye LA et al, The effect of pravastatin on coronary events after myocardial infarction in patients with average cholesterol levels, *N Engl J Med* 1996; **335**: 1001–9.

18. The Long-term Intervention with Pravastatin in Ischaemic Disease (LIPID) study group, prevention of cardiovascular events and death with pravastatin in patients with coronary heart disease and a broad range of initial cholesterol levels, *N Engl J Med* 1998; **339:** 1349–57.

19. Grundy SM, Statin trials and goals of cholesterol-lowering therapy, *Circulation* 1998; **97:** 1436–9.

20. Ericsson C-G, Hamsten A, Nilsson J, An angiographic evaluation of the effects of bezafibrate on the progression of coronary artery disease in young male post-infarction patients. The Bezafibrate Coronary Atherosclerosis Intervention Trial (BECAIT), *Lancet* 1996; **347:** 849–53.

21. Frick MH, Eli O, Haapa K, Heinonen OP, Heinsalmi P, Helo P, Helsinki Heart Study: primary-prevention trial with gemfibrozil in middle-aged men with dyslipidaemia. Safety of treatment, changes in risk factors, and incidence of coronary heart disease, *N Engl J Med* 1987; **317:** 1237–45.

22. MacMahon S, Peto R, Cutler J et al, Blood pressure, stroke and coronary heart disease: part 1, prolonged differences in blood pressure: prospective observational studies corrected for the regression dilution bias, *Lancet* 1990; **335:** 765–74.

23. Collins R, Peto R, MacMahon S et al, Blood pressure, stroke and coronary heart disease; part 2, short-term reductions in blood pressure: overview of randomised drug trials in their epidemiological context, *Lancet* 1990; **335:** 827–38.

24. Cutler JA, Psaty BM, MacMahon S, Furberg CD, Public health issues in hypertension control: what has been learned from clinical trials. In: Laragh JH, Brenner BM, eds, *Hypertension: Pathophysiology, Diagnosis and Management*, 2nd edn (Raven Press: New York, 1995) 253–70.

25. Hansson L, Zanchetti A, Carruthers SG et al, Effects of intensive blood-pressure lowering and low-dose aspirin in patients with hypertension: principal results of the Hypertension Optimal Treatment (HOT) randomised trial, *Lancet* 1998; **351:** 1755–62.

26. Yusuf S, Peto R, Lewis J, Collins R, Sleight P, Beta-blockade during and after myocardial infarction: an overview of the randomised trials, *Prog Cardiovasc Dis* 1985; **27:** 335–71.

27. Mcmurray J, *The ACE Inhibitor/Myocardial Infarction Trials* (Publishing Initiative Books: Beckenham, 1995).

28. Held PH, Yusuf S, Furberg CD, Calcium channel blockers in acute myocardial infarction and unstable angina: an overview, *Br Med J* 1989; **299:** 1187–92.

29. Stamler J, Vaccaro O, Neaton JD, Wentworth D, Diabetes, other risk factors, and 12-year cardiovascular mortality for men screened in the Multiple Risk Factor Intervention Trial, *Diabetes Care* 1993; **16:** 434–44.

30. The Diabetes Control and Complications Trial Research Group, The effect of intensive treatment of diabetes on the development and progression of long-term complications in insulin-dependent diabetes mellitus, *N Engl J Med* 1993; **329:** 977–86.

31. UK Prospective Diabetes Study (UKPDS) Group, Intensive blood-glucose control with sulphonylureas or insulin compared with conventional treatment and risk of complications in patients with type 2 diabetes (UKPDS 33), *Lancet* 1998; **352:** 837–53.

32. UK Prospective Diabetes Study (UKPDS) Group, Tight blood-pressure control and risk of macrovascular and microvascular

complications in type 2 diabetes (UKPDS 38), *Br Med J* 1998; **317**: 703–13.

33. Pyörälä K, Pedersen TR, Kjekshus J, Faergeman O, Olsson AG, Thorgeirsson G, Cholesterol lowering with simvastatin improves prognosis of diabetic patients with coronary heart disease, *Diabetes Care* 1997; **20**: 614–20.

34. Antiplatelet Trialists' Collaboration, Collaborative overview of randomised trials of antiplatelet therapy–1: prevention of death, myocardial infarction and stroke by prolonged antiplatelet therapy in various categories of patients, *Br Med J* 1994; **308**: 81–106.

35. CAPRIE Steering Committee, A randomised, blinded, trial of clopidogrel versus aspirin in patients at risk of ischaemic events (CAPRIE), *Lancet* 1996; **348**: 1329–39.

36. Grady D, Rubin SM, Petitti DB, Hormone therapy to prevent disease and prolong life in postmenopausal women, *Ann Intern Med* 1992; **117**: 1016–37.

37. Hulley S, Grady D, Bush T et al, Randomised trial of estrogen plus progestin for secondary prevention of coronary heart disease in postmenopausal women, *JAMA* 1998; **280**: 605–13.

38. Boushey CJ, Beresford SAA, Omenn GS, Motulsky AG, A quantitative assessment of plasma homocysteine as a risk factor for vascular disease. Probable benefits of increasing folic acid intakes, *JAMA* 1995; **274**: 1049–57.

39. Jha P, Flather M, Lonn E, Farkouh M, Yusuf S, Antioxidant vitamins and cardiovascular disease — a critical review of epidemiologic and clinical trial data, *Ann Intern Med* 1995; **123**: 860–72.

40. Stephens NG, Parsons A, Schofield PM et al, Randomised controlled clinical trial of vitamin E in patients with coronary disease: Cambridge Heart Antioxidant Study (CHAOS), *Lancet* 1996; **347**: 781–6.

41. Rapola JM, Virtamo J, Ripatti S et al, Randomised trial of alpha-tocopherol and beta-carotene supplements on incidence of major coronary events in men with previous myocardial infarction, *Lancet* 1997; **349**: 1715–20.

42. Rapola JM, Virtamo J, Ripatti S et al, Effects of α-tocopherol and β carotene supplements on symptoms, progression and prognosis of angina pectoris, *Heart* 1998; **79**: 454–8.

43. Weststrate JA, Meijer GW, Plant sterol enriched margarines and reduction of plasma total- and LDL-cholesterol concentrations in normocholesterolaemic and mildly hypercholesterolaemic subjects, *Eur J Clin Nut* 1998; **52**: 334–43.

44. EUROASPIRE Study Group, EUROASPIRE, A European Society of Cardiology survey of secondary prevention of coronary heart disease: principal results, *Eur Heart J* 1997; **18**: 1569–82.

Anti-anginal medication

Peter L Weissberg

4

Introduction

Patients develop the symptom of angina pectoris when
myocardial oxygenation is insufficient to satisfy demand.
Rarely, this is due to extreme oxygen demand in the context
of normal coronary bloodflow as, for example, in aortic
stenosis, where the remedy lies in correcting the mechanical
defect responsible for the excessive oxygen demand. However,
in most circumstances, angina is a manifestation of reduced
myocardial bloodflow due to coronary artery disease, where
medical therapy is directed at reducing myocardial demand or
increasing coronary bloodflow or both. To understand the
rationale behind different therapeutic approaches to the
management of angina, it is important to understand the
underlying vascular pathophysiology.

Traditionally, angina is described as being either stable or
unstable. In stable angina the symptoms are entirely
predictable and occur during recognized periods of increased
oxygen demand. In unstable angina the symptoms are
unpredictable, unprovoked or increasingly easily provoked.
The vascular pathology underlying these distinct syndromes is

different and will therefore be discussed before considering appropriate therapy.

The normal coronary artery

The normal coronary artery comprises a tube of vascular smooth muscle cells (the media) lined by a single layer of endothelial cells on the lumenal surface (the intima) and surrounded by loose connective tissue containing blood vessels (vasa vasora) and nerves (vasa nervora) on the outside (the adventitia). In the normal coronary artery the vascular smooth muscle cells contract and relax to alter the lumen diameter of the vessel in response to a variety of circulating and local stimuli. Over recent years it has become clear that the endothelium itself is one of the most important regulators of vascular smooth muscle tone via production of a number of vasoactive substances, including prostaglandins, vasoconstrictor peptides such as endothelin, and, most importantly, the endothelium-derived relaxing factor, now known to be the gas nitric oxide (NO), which as well as being a potent vasodilator is also an important endogenous inhibitor of platelet aggregation. It is now recognized that one of the earliest manifestations of atherosclerosis is abnormal endothelial function, in particular reduced NO production.[1]

The atherosclerotic plaque

Stable plaques

The earliest lesion in atherosclerosis is a subendothelial accumulation of lipid, known as a fatty streak. The persistence of lipid, particularly if oxidized, within the vessel wall initiates a local inflammatory reaction with activation of the overlying endothelial cells and recruitment of inflammatory cells, predominantly macrophages, into the subendothelial space, where they ingest oxidized lipid to become foam cells and produce a variety of cytokines. Some of these cytokines are chemoattractant and mitogenic for vascular smooth muscle cells and induce their migration from the vessel media into the intima, where they become incorporated into atherosclerotic lesion in the form of a cap overlying the lipid core (Fig. 4.1). Once in the intima, the smooth muscle cells lose their capacity to contract and gain the capacity to produce large amounts of collagenous and elastic extracellular matrix. Together, the intimal smooth muscle cells and their matrix form a protective fibrous cap over the lipid-rich atheromatous core.[2]

The fibrous cap is essential for the integrity of the plaque since the lipid core is highly thrombogenic and will readily induce local platelet aggregation and thrombosis if not isolated from the circulation by the cap. Furthermore, the collagenous nature of the fibrous cap is also thrombogenic and will attract and activate platelets if not itself protected by a layer of normally functioning endothelium. With time, the macrophage foam cells die and become incorporated into an enlarging necrotic lipid-rich core of the plaque. Thus lesions gradually increase in size at the expense of the vessel lumen until they limit flow enough to produce the symptom of stable angina when increased myocardial oxygen demand is not met. Provided the integrity of the endothelial surface and the fibrous cap remain intact, the angina is likely to be stable. Furthermore, lesions causing stable angina are characteristically large with a substantial fibrous cap and are readily visualized at angiography (Fig. 4.3).

Unstable plaques

Plaque instability occurs when the endothelium and/or fibrous cap overlying the lesion core become disrupted. The most important determinant of plaque stability is the balance between inflammatory cell activity and the healing, fibrotic action of the smooth muscle cells in the fibrous cap. If the inflammatory process gains the upper hand, there is destruction of the fibrous cap by a combination of direct cytotoxic effects of inflammatory cells on the smooth muscle cells in the cap and via production of enzymes, in particular matrix metalloproteinases, which degrade the matrix components of the cap.[2] The consequence of this inflammatory activity

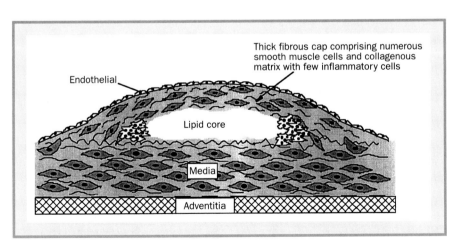

Figure 4.1
Stable atherosclerotic plaque.

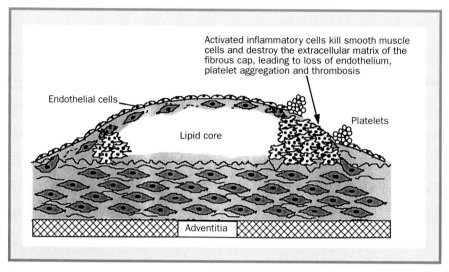

Activated inflammatory cells kill smooth muscle cells and destroy the extracellular matrix of the fibrous cap, leading to loss of endothelium, platelet aggregation and thrombosis

Endothelial cells

Platelets

Lipid core

Adventitia

Figure 4.2
Unstable atherosclerotic plaque.

is erosion of the cap and exposure of the underlying thrombogenic core to the circulation. This in turn leads to local platelet accumulation and activation, and, at its most extreme, thrombus formation and vessel occlusion. Thus, in contrast to the stable plaque, the unstable lesion is characterized by a thin fibrous cap, intense inflammatory activity and activation of thrombosis (Fig. 4.2).

Importantly, these features can and often are present in small, haemodynamically insignificant atherosclerotic plaques which

may not be apparent at angiography and may have previously been clinically silent (not causing stable angina).[3] Also, whereas stable angina is usually due to a fixed stenosis, release of vasoactive substances such as thromboxane A_2 and serotonin by activated platelets in unstable angina can provoke dynamic changes in local vascular tone which may contribute to symptoms (Fig. 4.3).

Thus the pathophysiological mechanisms underlying the development of stable and unstable angina are different. In stable angina the problem is one of mechanical limitation to

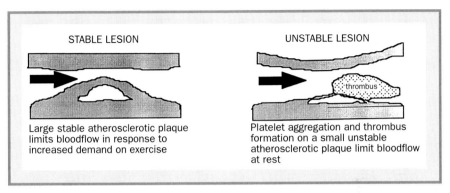

STABLE LESION

Large stable atherosclerotic plaque limits bloodflow in response to increased demand on exercise

UNSTABLE LESION

thrombus

Platelet aggregation and thrombus formation on a small unstable atherosclerotic plaque limit bloodflow at rest

Figure 4.3
Mechanism of stable and unstable angina.

coronary bloodflow, while in unstable angina the main problem is one of platelet aggregation and thrombosis; hence the approach to their management also differs. Recently, the term 'unstable coronary syndrome' has emerged and applies to clinical presentations of coronary disease in which plaque erosion or rupture is thought to be occurring. This term therefore encompasses myocardial infarction as well as unstable angina. However, with the advent of new sensitive and specific markers of myocardial damage, in particular circulating troponins, it is becoming clear that the distinction between myocardial infarction and unstable angina is less clearcut than was once thought, since patients with unstable angina and no ECG evidence of infarction will frequently have elevated troponin levels, indicating myocardial

damage.[4] The unstable coronary syndrome therefore represents a spectrum of thrombotic coronary disease encompassing, at one extreme, coronary occlusion and classical myocardial infarction, and at the other, minor endothelial erosions overlying small atherosclerotic plaques.

Medical management of stable angina

The objective of pharmacological management of stable angina is to improve the mismatch between myocardial oxygen supply and demand. Unlike skeletal muscle, which increases oxygen extraction from the blood during exercise, the myocardium undertakes maximum oxygen extraction at resting heart rates. Therefore, the only way of increasing oxygen supply to the myocardium is to increase coronary bloodflow, and inevitably if flow is limited by a fixed proximal lesion in a major coronary artery there is little scope for achieving this. Consequently, most anti-anginal therapies act by reducing oxygen demand.

Oxygen demand is determined by heart rate, contractility and myocardial wall stress, which is itself determined by end diastolic volume (preload) and outflow resistance (afterload).[5] Drugs which reduce any of these variables generally have an anti-anginal effect, whereas drugs which increase them (e.g. catecholamines) may precipitate angina. Of all the drugs which influence the cardiovascular system, three classes—nitrates, beta-adrenergic receptor antagonists and calcium channel blockers—have proven particularly effective in the management of stable angina and have been the mainstay of anti-anginal therapy for many years. A fourth class, potassium channel activators, has recently been added to this group, but experience with these drugs is limited.

Nitrates

Organic nitrates have been the mainstay of the management of angina for over a hundred years. They are converted to the vasoactive gas NO, which acts by increasing levels of cyclic GMP in vascular smooth muscle, which in turn regulates intracellular calcium to decrease vascular tone in coronary and peripheral arteries, and particularly in peripheral veins. Their effect on coronary arteries causes a temporary (few minutes) increase in coronary bloodflow, thereby increasing oxygen supply. However, their predominant and longer-lasting action is to reduce preload by venodilatation, thereby reducing oxygen demand.[6] This is countered to some extent by their tendency to lower blood pressure and induce reflex activation of the sympathetic nervous system. Nevertheless, overall, nitrates have a favourable effect on the oxygen supply/demand balance and are very effective anti-anginal agents.

Short-acting nitrates are taken both therapeutically to relieve angina when it is present, and prophylactically to prevent its onset during a specific physical task if taken immediately before beginning the task. For prompt relief of symptoms, glyceryl trinitrate (GTN 300–600 µg) is taken sublingually either as a tablet or as a metered aerosol. This is usually effective within 1–2 min and for up to 30 min. Because of its generalized vasodilating properties, GTN can cause transient hypotension, rarely leading to syncope, and often causes a headache. However, it is safe and can be taken repeatedly if necessary without serious toxicity. All patients with known coronary disease should carry and know how to use these short-acting nitrate preparations.

There are several oral preparations of longer-acting nitrates which are used for the chronic prophylaxis of angina, such as isosorbide dinitrate and isosorbide mononitrate, and slow-release preparations administered through the skin, 'nitrate patch' and GTN paste, or via the buccal mucosa. Each formulation reduces the frequency of angina attacks; however, a constant high plasma level of nitrates is undesirable because it induces tolerance.[7] Therefore, patients on long-acting nitrates are advised to have a nitrate-free period every 24 h, preferably overnight when their angina is less likely to be induced. Long-acting nitrates are generally well tolerated, with headache being the commonest side-effect. Patients who experience angina while taking a long-acting nitrate will usually still derive benefit from sublingual short-acting nitrates.

The value of nitrates is in their rapidity of action and lack of serious side-effects. However, there is no evidence that their use in angina has any effect on survival or morbidity.

Beta-adrenoreceptor antagonists (beta-blockers)

The predominant catecholamine receptor in the heart is the β_1 receptor, although there are some β_2 receptors in the myocardium and α and β_2 receptors in the coronary arteries. Stimulation of cardiac β_1 receptors causes an increase in heart rate (chronotropic effect) and an increase in force of contraction (inotropic effect), both of which increase myocardial oxygen demand. Beta-blockers therefore reduce heart rate and myocardial contractility at any given workload and thereby reduce oxygen demand. The supply/demand balance is further favourably influenced because they also reduce blood pressure (afterload) and, through their negative chronotropic effect, they prolong the diastolic period during which intramyocardial coronary bloodflow occurs. The negative chronotropic effect also leads to an increase in end diastolic volume and therefore wall tension. However, overall, beta-blockers have a favourable influence on the oxygen supply/demand balance and are very effective anti-anginal drugs.[8] They also abrogate the reflex sympathetic activity induced by nitrates, so the two classes of drug act synergistically.

β_1-Selective and non-selective beta-blockers are equally effective at preventing angina. The difference lies in their effects on other organs, in that β_1-selective blockers are less likely to cause bronchoconstriction and peripheral vasospasm than non-selective blockers. In rare instances, beta-blockers have been known to exacerbate angina. This is thought to be due to coronary vasospasm, theoretically induced by the unopposed action of catecholamines on coronary α receptors (coronary β_2 receptors mediate vasodilatation, while α receptors induce vasoconstriction). For this reason, beta-blockers should be used with caution in unstable coronary syndromes in which coronary vasospasm is thought to be playing a role. Despite their vasodilating properties, alpha-blockers have no role in the treatment of angina.

The main limitation to the use of beta-blockers in angina is their side-effects, most commonly a feeling of lethargy and cold extremities. More important side-effects include the onset or exacerbation of bronchospasm and deterioration in left ventricular function. The latter is more likely to occur when a beta-blocker is combined with another negative inotrope, such as calcium channel blocker (see below). Although there is no evidence that beta-blockers benefit outcome in patients with angina without previous myocardial infarction, they have been shown to reduce myocardial events and mortality if given during (intravenously) or following myocardial infarction.[9] Furthermore, recent studies have shown that, when appropriately administered, beta-blockers improve outcome in patients with heart failure.[10] They are therefore the obvious first choice anti-anginal in patients following myocardial infarction.

Calcium channel blockers

Calcium channel blockers reduce calcium influx into contractile cells. Therefore, in the heart they are negatively inotropic, whereas in coronary and peripheral arteries they reduce vascular tone. They have little effect on venous tone. The net effect is to reduce myocardial contractility and blood pressure (afterload) and increase coronary bloodflow, all of which have a favourable effect on the myocardial oxygen supply/demand balance. Some calcium channel blockers, in particular verapamil and to a lesser extent diltiazem, have an additional beneficial negative chronotropic effect. Although some short-acting calcium blockers, in particular nifedipine, are potent coronary vasodilators and may relieve acute angina, their tendency to reduce blood pressure and induce reflex sympathetic activity has called into question their use in acute coronary syndromes or following myocardial infarction, where they may be detrimental. Therefore, calcium channel blockers should generally be used only for the prophylaxis of angina in the form of slow-release or long-acting preparations. The one exception to this rule is in rare proven cases of Prinzemetal's variant angina in which short-acting nifedipine is very effective at reversing the coronary spasm causing the angina.[11]

Calcium channel blockers are a heterogeneous group of drugs with different therapeutic profiles. Dihydropyridines (nifedipine, amlodipine, nicardipine) have little effect on cardiac conduction, whereas verapamil (a phenylalkylamine) is a potent inhibitor of cardiac conduction, making it a useful anti-arrhythmic agent for supraventricular arrhythmias, but potentially dangerous in patients with inherent conduction disturbances, particularly when combined with beta-blockers. Diltiazem (a benzothiazepine) has a weak and generally unimportant effect on cardiac conduction.

Calcium channel blockers are generally well tolerated. The commonest side-effects include diuretic-resistant peripheral oedema (particularly the dihydropyridines), flushing (commonest with shorter-acting formulations), headache and constipation. Calcium channel blockers with potent negative inotropic properties, such as verapamil, should be avoided in patients with heart failure, particularly when combined with beta-blockers. As with nitrates, there is no evidence that use of calcium channel blockers for the treatment of angina confers any outcome benefit.

Potassium channel activators

This is a relatively new class of anti-anginal drug of which nicorandil is the prototype. By increasing potassium flux across smooth muscle cell membranes, it causes vasodilatation. Nicorandil shares many properties with nitrates, but without inducing tolerance. It is therefore a suitable substitute for long-acting nitrates in the treatment of angina and may also be used in combination with any or all of the above classes of anti-anginal drugs. Experience with nicorandil is still somewhat limited and its place in the management of angina remains to be established. Side-effects are few and similar to those of nitrates, predominantly headache. However, it is not negatively inotropic and does not induce bronchospasm. Therefore, it may be used in patients with impaired cardiac function or asthma in whom calcium channel blockers and beta-blockers may be contraindicated. It is also possible that potassium channel openers may protect the heart from ischaemic damage.[12] This is because it has been found in experimental models that a short-lived ischaemic event protects the heart from damage during a second, more prolonged, ischaemic event, a phenomenon known as ischaemic preconditioning, and activation of potassium channels is an essential feature of ischaemic preconditioning. Further research is required to determine if this theoretical benefit is realized in clinical practice.

Combination therapy

Members of the above classes of drugs can be used alone or combined with members of other classes, such that it is acceptable and indeed sometimes desirable for some patients

Table 4.1
Mechanisms of anti-anginal drug action.

	Nitrates	Beta- blockers	Ca²⁺ channel blockers	K⁺ channel openers	Combination
Heart rate	↑^{a}	↓	↓↑	↑^{a}	↓
Blood pressure	↓	↓	↓	↓	↓↓^{b}
LV wall tension	↓	↑	↓	↓	↓
LV contractility	↑^{a}	↓^{c}	↓^{c}	↑^{a}	↓^{c}
Coronary flow	↑	↑	↑	↑	↑

^{a}Via reflex sympathetic activity. ^{b}Risk of hypotension when combined. ^{c}Risk of heart failure.

to be receiving nitrates, a beta-blocker, a calcium channel blocker and possibly also nicorandil (Table 4.1). However, in most instances patients with drug-resistant angina would be considered for non-pharmacological therapy such as angioplasty or coronary bypass surgery before receiving full combined therapy. Opinion varies as to which is the most appropriate first-line anti-anginal drug, and therapy should be tailored towards the needs of individual patients and is often dictated by the presence of other conditions such as hypertension, heart failure or asthma.

Medical management of unstable angina

The syndrome of unstable angina is caused by erosion or rupture of often small

atherosclerotic lesions with subsequent platelet aggregation, thrombosis and vasospasm leading to reduced coronary perfusion and myocardial ischaemia. The objectives of therapy in unstable angina are therefore to reverse the prothrombotic environment in the coronary artery, as well as to relieve symptoms.

Nitrates

Nitrates are used in unstable angina to relieve symptoms. As discussed above, their main mode of action is to reduce preload and therefore oxygen demand. However, in unstable angina it is probable that nitrates also counter the local vasoconstrictive effects of platelet products such as thromboxane A$_2$ and serotonin, such that their coronary vasodilating properties are probably more important in unstable than in stable angina.[13] The commonest method of nitrate administration in unstable angina is in the form of a GTN or isosorbide dinitrate infusion of 1–10 mg/h. Because of its short half-life (2–3 min), the dose can be readily titrated against the patient's symptoms or side-effects, the commonest of which are headache and hypotension. An alternative, though less flexible, method of chronic nitrate therapy in unstable angina is the use of different strengths of buccal nitrate tablets which can be discarded or changed according to symptoms or side-effects. Nitrate infusions may be continued for several days, albeit at the risk of inducing tolerance.

Antiplatelet drugs

Drugs which inhibit platelet aggregation are a logical choice and have proven benefit in the treatment of unstable angina.[14] For many years, acetylsalicylic acid (aspirin) was, and in most coronary care units still is, the mainstay of antiplatelet therapy in unstable angina. Aspirin irreversibly inhibits the platelet cyclo-oxygenase responsible for prostaglandin production, and at low doses (75–150 mg daily) preferentially inhibits thromboxane A_2 production and therefore platelet aggregation. However, aspirin's effects on prostaglandins are not confined to platelets; hence its high incidence of gastrointestinal side-effects, even

at low dosage. Therefore, over recent years, with increasing knowledge of platelet biology, there has been a rapid expansion in the development of drugs designed specifically to inhibit platelet aggregation and activity. In addition to aspirin, the antiplatelet armamentarium now includes agents such as dipyridamole, ticlopidine, clopidogrel and a variety of glycoprotein IIb/IIIa antagonists.[15]

Dipyridamole is an inhibitor of platelet phosphodiesterase and is also a potent vasodilatory which can at times exacerbate angina by diverting blood away from the ischaemic area (coronary steal syndrome). Therefore, it is not indicated for the management of unstable angina. Ticlopidine and clopidogrel are ADP receptor antagonists that inhibit platelet binding to fibrin. Ticlopidine has been extensively used to prevent thrombotic occlusion following insertion of coronary stents and it has been shown in clinical trials to be beneficial in unstable angina. However, in up to 3% of patients it induces serious neutropenia, which, although usually reversible if the drug is stopped, can sometimes be fatal. Clopidogrel is a derivative of ticlopidine that does not appear to induce neutropenia. It has recently been shown to prevent cardiovascular events in patients with previous vascular disease,[16] but its effects in unstable angina have yet to be formally evaluated.

The glycoprotein IIb/IIIa integrin is responsible for crosslinking platelets to each other and to fibrin and represents the final common pathway in platelet aggregation, regardless of the stimulus to platelet activation. A variety of antagonists, including monoclonal antibodies, and synthetic peptide and non-peptide inhibitors, for systemic and oral administration have been developed. They are potent antiplatelet agents and those that have been tested in unstable angina have been shown to be of benefit.[17] However, the risk of haemorrhage is substantial when they are combined with heparin, and further research is required to establish their role in unstable angina.

There are numerous clinical trials of a variety of antiplatelet agents currently underway in unstable coronary syndromes, and the coming years are likely to see considerable changes in their use based on results from these trials. Suffice it to say that in unstable coronary syndromes antiplatelet therapy is mandatory, and all patients with unstable angina should receive aspirin 75–150 mg daily unless specifically contraindicated, in which case an alternative antiplatelet drug should be considered. On today's evidence, clopidogrel would seem to be an appropriate choice.[16]

Antithrombotic therapy

Heparin enhances the capacity of endogenous antithrombin III to inhibit thrombin and activated factor X (Xa), the first protein in the final common pathway to coagulation via both the intrinsic and extrinsic pathways. It is a potent anticoagulant with proven benefit in the management of unstable angina.[14] Until recently it was available only as an unfractionated mixture of purified heparins of varying molecular weight. Because of the heterogeneous nature of these preparations, their anticoagulant action has to be monitored in the laboratory and the dose adjusted according to the activated partial thromboplastin time (APTT) in each individual. Because heparin is poorly absorbed, it has to be given systemically either as an intravenous infusion or subcutaneously. Most heparinization regimens involve an initial intravenous bolus of 5000 units followed by an infusion of 1000–2000 units per hour, adjusted after 6 h according to the APTT result. Inadequate anticoagulation is ineffective, while over-anticoagulation increases the risk of haemorrhagic complications.

Over recent years, several low molecular weight heparins have been developed with equivalent anticoagulant activity to unfractionated heparin and a much more predictable therapeutic effect, such that, provided the appropriate dose is given (based on the patient's weight), there is no need to monitor the anticoagulant effect. Furthermore, low molecular weight heparins can be administered as a single or twice-daily subcutaneous injection. Recent studies have demonstrated that these preparations are at least as effective as unfractionated heparins in the treatment of unstable angina.[18] The main obstacle to their widespread adoption as routine therapy for unstable angina is their cost, which is substantially greater than that of unfractionated heparin. However, economic assessments are beginning to demonstrate that when ease of administration and cost of infusion pumps and therapeutic monitoring are taken into account, the argument in favour of low molecular weight heparin is strengthened.

The main risk of heparin therapy is bleeding, which can occur spontaneously or at sites of previous trauma or pathology. Because of its short half-life, most bleeding problems can be dealt with by stopping the infusion or, if necessary, the anticoagulant effect of heparin can be reserved by protamine sulphate. A much rarer, though serious, complication of heparin therapy is heparin-induced thrombocytopoenia. This is an immunological reaction to heparin which can lead to widespread thrombosis. Fortunately, it usually only occurs in patients receiving heparin for more than a week and is therefore rarely a problem in patients receiving heparin for unstable angina.

Although, intuitively, thrombolytic agents might be expected to be of benefit in unstable angina, this has proven not to be the case in randomized clinical trials. There is therefore no place for thrombolysis in the management of unstable angina.

In summary, therefore, patients with unstable angina should receive aspirin or an alternative antiplatelet agent and should receive nitrates and heparin for the duration of their symptoms. Addition of beta-blockers will often provide further symptomatic benefit. Traditionally, nitrate and heparin therapy are continued until cardiac pain has been absent for at least 24 h. Thereafter, aspirin should be continued indefinitely, and conventional oral anti-anginal therapy can be substituted for systemic nitrates, if required.

Because unstable angina is frequently caused by erosion of a haemodynamically insignificant atherosclerotic plaque, once the unstable symptoms have resolved the patient may remain angina-free. However, a substantial proportion of patients presenting with unstable angina will go on to experience recurrent episodes of either stable or unstable angina or will be refractory to medical therapy and will require investigation with a view to intervention to improve their coronary circulation.

Secondary prevention

Patients with stable or unstable angina, by definition, have coronary artery disease and are therefore at substantial risk of a cardiovascular event. Their presentation therefore provides an opportunity to modify their cardiac risk factors, such as smoking habit, diet and hypertension, and to institute therapy to prevent further cardiac events. There is now strong evidence that all patients with coronary artery disease should be prescribed daily aspirin 75–150 mg[19] (it is currently not known whether other antiplatelet agents will have the same long-term cardioprotective effects as aspirin); a statin if their cholesterol remains elevated above 4 mmol/l after appropriate dietary advice (large outcome studies with pravastatin and simvastatin have demonstrated impressive protection against future cardiac events, possibly by enhancing stability of pre-existing atherosclerotic plaques);[20,21] a beta-blocker if they have experienced a previous myocardial infarction;[9] and an angiotensin-converting enzyme inhibitor if they have impaired left ventricular function.[22]

References

1. Ross R, Atherosclerosis—an inflammatory disease, *N Engl J Med* 1999; **340**(2): 115–26.

2. Libby P, Molecular bases of the acute coronary syndromes, *Circulation* 1995; **91**: 2844–50.

3. Falk E, Fuster V, Angina-pectoris and disease progression, *Circulation* 1995; **92**(8): 2033–5.

4. Stubbs P, The cardiac troponins: uses in routine clinical practice—experiences from

GUSTO and other clinical trials, *Eur Heart J* 1998; **19**: N59–63.

5. Braunwald E, Sobel B, Coronary blood flow and myocardial ischaemia. In: Braunwald E, ed., *Heart Disease: a Textbook of Cardiovascular Medicine*, 4th edn (WB Saunders: Philadelphia, 1992) 1161–99.

6. Parker J, Nitrate therapy in stable angina pectoris, *N Engl J Med* 1987; **316**: 1635–42.

7. Colditz G, Halvorsen K, Goldhaber S, Randomized clinical trials of transdermal nitroglycerin systems for the treatment of chronic stable angina: a meta-analysis, *Am Heart J* 1998; **116**: 174–80.

8. Rutherford J, Braunwald E, Chronic ischaemic heart disease. In: Braunwald E, ed., *Heart Disease: a Textbook of Cardiovascular Medicine*, 4th edn (WB Saunders: Philadelphia, 1992) 1292–381.

9. Yusuf S. Peto R, Lewis J, Collins R, Sleight P, Beta blockade during and after myocardial infarction: an overview of the randomized trials, *Prog Cardiovasc Dis* 1985; **27**: 335–71.

10. Lechat P, Packer M, Chalon S, Cucherat M, Arab T, Biossel J, Clinical effects of beta adrenergic blockade in chronic heart failure— a meta-analysis of double-blind, placebo-controlled, randomized trials, *Circulation* 1998; **98**: 1184–91.

11. Antman E, Muller J, Goldberg S et al, Nifedipine therapy for coronary-artery spasm. Experience in 127 patients, *N Engl J Med* 1980; **302**: 12–16.

12. Imagawa J, Baxter G, Yellon D, Myocardial protection afforded by nicorandil and ischaemic preconditioning in rabbit infarct model in vivo, *J Cardiovasc Pharmacol* 1998; **31**: 74–9.

13. Willerson J, Golino P, Eidt J, Campbell W, Buja J, Specific platelet mediators and unstable coronary artery lesions. Experimental

evidence and potential clinical implications, *Circulation* 1989; **80**: 198–205.

14. Theroux P, Ouimet H, McCans J et al, Aspirin, heparin, or both to treat unstable angina, *N Engl J Med* 1988; **313**: 1105–11.

15. White H, French J, Ellis C, New antiplatelet agents, *Aus NZ J Med* 1998; **28**: 558–64.

16. CAPRIE Steering Committee, A randomised, blinded, trial of clopidogrel versus aspirin in patients at risk of ischaemic events (CAPRIE), *Lancet* 1996; **348**(9038): 1329–39.

17. Alexander J, Harrington R, Recent antiplatelet drug trials in the acute coronary syndromes— clinical interpretation of PRISM, PRISM-PLUS, PARAGON A and PURSUIT, *Drugs* 1998; **56**: 965–76.

18. Cohen M, Demers C, Gurfinkel E et al, A comparison of low-molecular-weight heparin with unfractionated heparin for unstable coronary artery disease, *N Engl J Med* 1997; **337**: 447–52.

19. ATP Collaboration. Secondary prevention of vascular disease by prolonged antiplatelet treatment. *Br Med J* 1988; **296**: 320–31.

20. Scandinavian Simvastatin Survival Group, Randomised trial of cholesterol lowering in 4444 patients with coronary heart disease: the Scandinavian Simvastatin Survival Study (4S), *Lancet* 1994; **344**: 1383–9.

21. Lipid Study Group, Prevention of cardiovascular events and death with pravastatin in patients with coronary heart disease and a broad range of initial cholesterol levels, *N Engl J Med* 1998; **339**(19): 1349–57.

22. Ball S, Hall A, Who should be treated with angiotensin converting enzyme inhibitors after myocardial infarction? *Am Heart J* 1996; **132**(1): 244–50.

Coronary arteriography

David L Stone

The advent of coronary arteriography revolutionized the field of diagnostic cardiology. Catheterization of the left side of the heart was first described in the early 1950s by Zimmerman et al.[1] However, it was not until selective coronary arteriography was reported in 1959 by Mason Sones that the clinical implications began to be realized. In the 1960s, work by Rickets and Abrams[2] described percutaneous techniques for performing cine arteriography of the coronary arterial tree, and Judkins[3] developed the first pre-shaped catheters.

The development of a technique that could provide precise anatomical information about the arteries to the heart, paralleling the application of bypass grafting to the coronary vessels, opened the door to an interventional approach to cardiology which superseded the more conventional tablet-based treatments available at that time.

Indications

The indications for coronary arteriography are:

- to define the extent and position of obstructive coronary

arterial lesions in patients thought to have angina pectoris based on symptoms and exercise testing;

- to confirm or refute the presence of coronary arterial disease in patients presenting with atypical symptoms and/or investigations;
- to monitor the progress of arterial disease post-transplantation;
- to identify coronary arterial disease in patients undergoing surgery for other cardiac pathology, e.g. aortic stenosis.

These indications may well define the broad applications of coronary arteriography, but the timing of the investigation during the course of disease progression is much more problematic and requires considerable skill and experience on the part of the clinician. In any individual case, much will depend upon availability of facilities, expertise and funding, all of which inform local attitudes and practices. Guidelines are often centrally issued, for example in the USA by the American College of Cardiology.[4] In the UK, where waiting lists are ubiquitous, there is also a need to prioritize cases according to perceived risk. There is considerable debate as to how exactly this should be achieved. Imposed guidelines for healthcare may set arbitrary targets (1000 procedures/year per million population in the author's locality) which fail to take into account individual cases, with the result that the responsibility for waiting list

management often falls to the individual cardiologist. In the author's unit, a system of consensus guidelines has been adopted, whereby the local cardiologists and cardiac surgeons jointly agree evidence-based policies (where possible) with regard to patient selection and prioritization.

The current criteria are:

- limiting angina despite at least one anti-anginal medication;
- post-myocardial infarction with evidence of ongoing ischaemia as determined by symptoms of angina pectoris and/or positive exercise test or perfusion scan;
- patients over the age of 40 years undergoing valve surgery;
- to determine the presence or absence of coronary arterial disease in patients with multiple admissions with chest pain.

Priority is given to:

- patients with a very positive exercise test (less than 6 min of Standard Bruce Protocol, extensive ST segment change, significant fall in blood pressure);
- unstable angina;
- social reasons, e.g. occupation at risk, sole carer.

Other situations in which arteriography may be *considered* include:

- any patient under the age of 50 years having suffered a myocardial infarction;
- patients with positive exercise test results post-myocardial infarction but few or no symptoms;
- patients with known angina pectoris awaiting major elective surgery for non-cardiac conditions, e.g. total hip replacement;
- young patients (under 60 years) presenting with heart failure of unknown cause.

Procedure

As with any surgical procedure, the patient's informed consent is obtained prior to the administration of pre-medication, if required. In the author's unit, it is current practice to prescribe 10–15 mg diazepam for patients anticipating an overnight stay in hospital. Many centres now offer cardiac catheterization as a day-case procedure, and pre-medication is usually omitted in these patients, in order that they may be discharged without unnecessary delay.

The first step for the operator is to gain vascular access. To ensure a smooth, successful procedure with the minimum discomfort and risk of local damage, the optimum site for arterial puncture must be selected. This depends upon both the history and examination, with the operator paying particular attention to symptoms and signs of possible peripheral

vascular disease, such as intermittent claudication, femoral bruits or absence of foot pulses. The three most commonly selected arterial sites for cannulation are:

- femoral
- brachial
- radial

Having selected, prepared and draped the site, the operator then chooses to approach the vessel either percutaneously or by cut-down. The latter is used for the brachial artery only.

Percutaneous approach

This technique has changed little since it was originally described by Seldinger in 1953.[5] The skin and subcutaneous tissues overlying the chosen vessel are infiltrated with local anaesthetic, e.g. 10 ml lignocaine 1%. A 1–2 mm incision is made in the skin using a number 11 scalpel blade. The artery is punctured by a hollow, narrow-gauge needle. A guidewire with a soft flexible tip is passed through the needle and advanced a short way into the vessel, ensuring that little or no resistance is encountered. If the wire does not move freely, it should be gently withdrawn and another attempt made. *The operator must never attempt to force the wire into the vessel against resistance.* Indeed, if it is felt that the vessel is or may be damaged, the needle should be withdrawn completely along with the wire and firm pressure applied to the site for 2–4 min before repeat puncture is attempted.

Once the wire is in place, the needle is withdrawn over it and a valved sheath passed over the wire into the vessel. The wire is them removed and the sidearm of the sheath is flushed with normal saline.

The specially pre-shaped catheters can now be introduced and advanced via the arterial system into the aortic root in order to selectively cannulate, under fluoroscopic screening, the ostia of the right and left coronary arteries. The X-ray tube is rotated about the patient in order to obtain multiple views of each vessel; 3–10 ml non-ionic contrast medium is injected for each view. After coronary arteriography, a catheter with multiple holes near the tip (usually a 'pigtail' catheter) is passed through the aortic valve into the left ventricular cavity. Pressure measurements may be made and a left ventriculogram performed by injecting 20–35 ml non-ionic contrast medium using a mechanical injecting device. This produces a characteristic 'hot flush' about which the patient should be warned.

At the end of the procedure, the catheter is removed and the sheath also.

Following the removal of the sheath, firm pressure is applied to the puncture site for a period of 5–15 min, or sometimes even longer, until the bleeding has stopped. This part of the procedure is of critical importance in terms of local bleeding complications. In many centres, trained nurses are successfully performing this manoeuvre. The patient is then asked to press on the site until transferred back to the ward. There is then a period of bed rest, of approximately 3 h.

The patient is then mobilized and may be allowed to go home later in the day. The percutaneous technique is sometimes used for the brachial artery approach. For this, the left brachial is easier. The technique is identical, although choice of catheters is different. The patient may be mobilized immediately.

Another approach is via the radial artery. Although allowing very early mobilization, this is more painful[6] and the catheters are more difficult to manoeuvre.

All techniques provide diagnostic-quality angiograms.

A typical catheter laboratory is shown in Fig. 5.1 and the manifold for contrast injection and pressure measurement in Fig. 5.2.

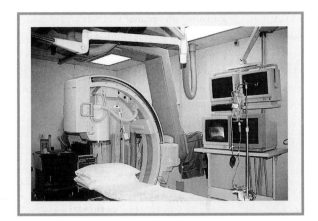

Figure 5.1
Photograph of typical cardiac catheter laboratory.

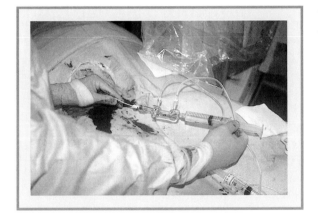

Figure 5.2
Injection manifold. This allows easy pressure measurement and injection of contrast.

Approach by cut-down

This technique was proposed by Stones et al[7] and is used for the right brachial artery primarily. Preparation is the same as for the femoral route. Following infiltration of local anaesthetic, an incision of about 3 cm in length is made over the brachial artery. Blunt dissection is used to expose the brachial artery, and tapes are placed around it. The vessel is then lifted and a 1–2 mm incision made directly into it (some operators insert a sheath at this point) and the catheters are passed through the incision around the aorta until the aortic root is reached and from then the angiographic part of the procedure is similar to that described above.

Once the procedure is complete, the catheter is removed and the artery sewn up by direct suture, usually using fine prolene. The skin incision is then sutured with nylon or silk. The radial pulse is palpated following the procedure. Mobilization may be immediate. Although this technique has many supporters, most operators prefer the femoral Seldinger technique which is easier to learn.

Findings

Coronary arteriography defines the anatomy of the coronary vessels and the lesions within them. It does not provide functional information, for which exercise testing, whether it be assessed by ECG, perfusion scintigraphy or radionuclide ventriculography, is required. The site and extent of lesions have nevertheless been related to prognosis.[8,9]

Anatomy

There are two main coronary arteries, left and right. The left main stem is the term applied to that portion of the left coronary that is proximal to its division into the left anterior descending and left circumflex branches. The anterior descending is situated in the anterior interventricular sulcus and supplies branches into the interventricular septum and diagonal branches to the superolateral portion of the left ventricle. The circumflex vessel descends in the posterior atrioventricular sulcus to supply obtuse marginal branches to the posterolateral wall of the left ventricle.

The right coronary falls in the anterior atrioventricular sulcus to supply right ventricular branches, which do not have clinical significance, and the posterior descending vessel and inferior left ventricular branches, which do. The vessel which gives the posterior descending vessel is said to be 'dominant'. In 90% of cases that is the right, and in 10% the left. If the left is dominant, the whole of the left ventricular blood supply comes from that vessel.

Angiography, as has been seen, may be performed in the investigation of chronic angina pectoris or in the acute situation after infarction.

Coronary arteriography in chronic angina

By far the most widespread application of the technique of coronary arteriography has been in patients with chronic stable angina. The indications used in our centre have already been discussed. The lesions are generally assessed in clinical practice by visual analysis. The use of multiple projections allows better judgement of individual lesions as well as exposing narrowings which are only seen in one view, either because of overlapping of vessels or because the lesion itself is eccentric in position within any given vessel.

There have been computerized methods developed which enable more objective scoring of lesions by wall detection algorithms. Although popular in experimental situations, they appear to confer little benefit in day-to-day practice.

There is also much debate about what constitutes a 'significant' lesion. Often, the decision about intervention rests on whether a lesion occupies at least 50% of luminal diameter, judged visually. This is a rough estimate in any case and lesions as little as 30% have been shown in the experimental situation to cause metabolically important restriction of flow,[10] which was not seen in the resting state. Nonetheless, the 50% level has been accepted widely and is, indeed, widely applied.

It should be pointed out that a truer assessment would be obtained by combining clinical, angiographic and functional information, e.g. from radionuclide perfusion studies. This has become all the more important since the advent of angioplasty in virtually all angiography centres. It is all too easy to make a decision based on the anatomical angiographic findings without taking into account symptoms or functional information which provides objective evidence of ischaemia. Certainly, if there is a disparity between symptoms and angiography, then these techniques must be employed to complement the arteriography.

Since extent of disease defines prognosis, a common description of coronary narrowing is of one-, two- or three-vessel disease. This is a shorthand way of describing the overall spread of narrowing. Although convenient, it gives no indication as to whether the lesions are proximal or distal. Proximal disease subtends more myocardium and is therefore potentially more dangerous. Coronary scoring systems have been devised but have little place in current clinical practice. Information may also be gleaned about the nature of the individual lesions and their extent and complexity. The shape of the arterial tree is defined.

All these data allow the operator to decide upon whether angioplasty is feasible, which it may not be, even in patients with less extensive disease normally considered for this intervention.

The final clinical decision must be based on all

these factors. The aim of any revascularization procedure is to improve symptoms. Nonetheless, prognostic benefit is accrued in certain anatomical situations. In the studies mentioned previously, bypass surgery offered prognostic benefit in patients with left main stem stenosis (a lesion in the main stem of the left coronary before its division into anterior descending and circumflex branches), and those with triple-vessel disease and impaired left ventricular function. The information from angiography guides treatment choices but must not be the only arbiter.

Acute situation

In the acute situation, information is most needed with respect to the anatomy of the lesion responsible for the specific problem. Of course, anatomical information about the other vessels as well as left ventricular function is also obtained. The type of lesion, its site and the presence of associated thrombus or dissection are demonstrated. On the basis of this, a clinical decision must be made as to whether it would be appropriate to proceed to an intervention, angioplasty or operation or to continue medical management. The patient's clinical situation is assessed and related to the site and nature of the obstruction. The presence of excessive thrombus or arterial tortuosity might make angioplasty hazardous. The finding of multiple coronary lesions may mean that surgery is indicated.

Catheterization in aortic stenosis

Angina may occur in aortic stenosis and require investigation by catheterization, especially in the over-40 age group.

The procedure is similar to routine coronary arteriography but the aortic valve may be difficult to cross to measure the pressure drop at peak systole. An aortogram is performed to quantify degree of aortic regurgitation and size of aortic root. The coronary vessels are difficult to cannulate due to distortion and enlargement of the aortic root, and sometimes to the origins of the coronary vessels are aberrant, presumably associated with a congential bicuspid valve. The investigations are among the most difficult technically and should not be undertaken by inexperienced operators. It is not essential in these patients to perform a left ventriculogram during the procedure, as the information may be obtained from echocardiogram or radionuclide ventriculogram

Examples

In order to demonstrate the kind of findings obtained at arteriography, I have included illustrations of typical cases (Figs 5.3–5.8).

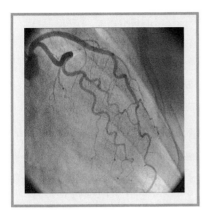

Figure 5.3
Normal left coronary artery.

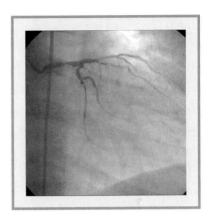

Figure 5.5
Tight lesion in main stem of left coronary artery. The lesion is seen prior to the division of the left coronary artery into the anterior descending and circumflex vessels.

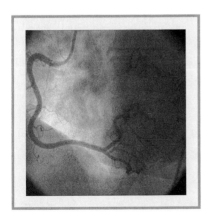

Figure 5.4
Normal right coronary artery.

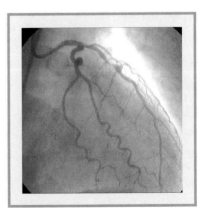

Figure 5.6
Tight stenosis of the left anterior descending artery.

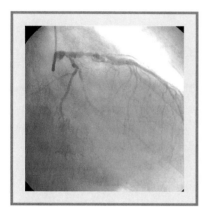

Figure 5.7
Severe left coronary artery disease involving
anterior descending and circumflex vessels.

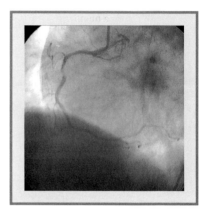

Figure 5.8
Tight narrowing of proximal right coronary artery
with associated thrombus.

Complications

Cardiac catheterization is an invasive
procedure. As such, complications must be
expected to occur. In a major study of
complications of catheterization,
complications occurred in 1.74% of all
patients.[11]

The complication rate is related to the
experience of the operator to an important
extent. Any training cardiologist must have
careful supervision from the outset. Bad habits
or a lackadaisical attitude create continued
problems and put patients at risk. The
operator also may lose confidence, which has
an ongoing detrimental effect.

The major complications may be categorized
as:

• local arterial damage
• cardiac
• extracardiac
• death

Local arterial damage

When the femoral Seldinger technique is
used, the most common local complications
are groin haematoma, false aneurysm,
arteriovenous fistula, and arterial dissection.
Bruising is almost universal and the patient
should be warned that the blood may track
down to the knee.

Many of the problems may be averted by careful technique during the procedure and careful attention to detail during the groin pressure following removal of the sheath. If false aneurysm is suspected, radiological advice with respect to ultrasound should be sought. A surgical opinion should be obtained early. All aspects of the management must be documented fully in the patient's notes, as litigation may take place. Local dissection does not necessitate intervention but if the limb is threatened or there is an expanding aneurysm then open repair is indicated.

With the brachial approach there may be complete occlusion of the artery, which is identified by loss of pulse at the wrist and a cold, ischaemic hand. Again, the key to a successful outcome is early involvement of the surgeon, with appropriate repair if necessary.

Arterial complications occur in 0.6–1% of catheterizations.[12]

Cardiac complications

These are:

- arrhythmias
- conduction disturbances
- myocardial infarction

Arrhythmias

Major arrythmias requiring therapy occur in about 0.5% of patients. Ventricular tachycardia and fibrillation occurred in 0.54% of patients in one reported series.[13]

It is obvious that a defibrillator must be present at all coronary arteriography procedures. Short episodes of ventricular tachycardia are common, particularly when the catheter is lying against the wall of the ventricle. More prolonged episodes are more common in severely ischaemic patients or if the catheter is not removed from the wall of the ventricle and injection of contrast medium takes place. Ventricular fibrillation may be avoided by using the minimum amount of contrast medium and avoiding injecting, even by hand, when a side-branch of the artery, usually the right coronary, has been entered. However, the ventricular fibrillation usually responds quickly to DC shock. The use of non-ionic contrast media has significantly reduced the incidence of these arrythmias.

Atrial arrhythmias are more common during right heart catheterization. Nonetheless, they may occur during coronary arteriography. Again, they usually settle quickly. Marked sinus bradycardia and hypotension are usually due to vasovagal reactions related to the arterial puncture in anxious patients or those having pain. The bradycardia usually precedes the hypotension and is associated with sweating. The treatment is rapid administration of 0.6–1.2 mg of intravenous atropine and fluid replacement if necessary.

Conduction disturbances

Complete heart block is extremely uncommon after left heart catheterization, even in patients with pre-existing bundle branch block. The incidence has fallen even further with the use of non-ionic media. Prophylactic temporary pacemakers need not therefore be inserted during diagnostic angiography.

Myocardial infarction

The incidence of myocardial infarction appears to be around 1%. Predisposing factors include: instability of the angina being investigated, recent infarction and left main stem stenosis. Mechanisms that may be responsible are myocardial hypoperfusion, untreated and ongoing ischaemia and coronary embolism. Prophylactic insertion of an intra-aortic balloon pump in very unstable patients may prove very beneficial, especially if further intervention is being contemplated.

Extracardiac complications
Neurological

The most worrying neurological complication of cardiac catheterization is stroke. This has been shown to occur in 0.07% of cases,[11,14] and is independent of the technique used. It is nearly always embolic, and can be shown to be so by computed tomography or magnetic resonance imaging of the brain. Emboli may be due to thrombus, cholesterol or air. They may be prevented by meticulous attention to detail during the procedure. All guidewires must be carefully wiped. Advancement of the catheter around the arch must be gentle, and the floppy end of the guidewire must be leading the way. Entry into the brachiocephalic trunks should be avoided, especially in elderly patients.

Migraine is common immediately after the procedure, particularly in known sufferers. Other rare neurological complications are spinal cord embolization, seizures and cortical blindness.

Renal complications

These occur in about 0.23%[11] and may be due to direct nephrotoxicity of the contrast medium or emboli to the kidneys. Risk factors are evidence of previous renal impairment and diabetes. Large volumes of contrast medium should be avoided. Patients at risk should be adequately hydrated for the procedure. Severe renal impairment is rare, but minor changes are common and often not appreciated.

Infection and febrile reactions

Both febrile reactions and bacteraemia are now rare. Antibiotic prophylaxis in valve cases is therefore not recommended.

Attention to antiseptic technique, is of course, vital.

Death

The death of the patient is the most feared complication of diagnostic catheterization. It is all the more distressing because neither operator nor patient nor often the patient's family expects it during what is essentially an investigative rather than a therapeutic procedure. Death occurs in about 0.1% of procedures.[11,14] Death is more common in patients over the age of 65, those with left main stem disease, and those with heart failure with or without documented reduction in ejection fraction.

It should not be anticipated that the incidence of death at catheterization will fall, since more unstable and ill patients are being investigated, especially in the angioplasty era. A major avenue to improve safety is in the patient with suspected left main stem stenosis. If such a lesion is seen, the cannula tip must be kept away from the stenosis and an absolute minimum of views of the coronary vessels obtained. It must never be forgotten that the aim of the procedure is to obtain diagnostic information, sufficient to guide as accurately as possible future management. It is *not* to obtain artistically perfect images. If the lesion is suspected before the procedure, for example if there is a very positive exercise test at low workload, then an anteroposterior view should be taken first, as this allows clear visualization of the main stem.

It is vitally important that the operator speaks to the relatives immediately after the death to explain the situation.

Conclusions

Coronary arteriography has driven cardiology forwards at a remarkable rate. The ability to provide diagnostically critical information at minimal risk has allowed other techniques such as cardiac surgery and percutaneous angioplasty to flourish. Also, the practising clinician can be confident that the information obtained is accurate and is able to give better prognostic advice. This confidence transfers to the patients and creates a positive dynamic approach to the management of such ubiquitous and dangerous disease. Other techniques have threatened to displace it from the scene, such as magnetic resonance imaging but the technical difficulties of accessing accurate data from the moving heart have not allowed sufficient resolution to displace a procedure that may be performed on relatively standard X-ray equipment found in most departments.

References

1. Zimmerman HA, Scott RW, Becker ND, Catheterisation of the left side of the heart in man, *Circulation* 1950; **1**: 357–9.

2. Ricketts JH, Abrams HL, Percutaneous selective coronary cine arteriography, *JAMA* 1962; **181**: 620–4.

3. Judkins MP, Selective coronary arteriography: a percutaneous transfemoral technique, *Radiology* 1967; **89**: 815–24.

4. Pepine CJ, Allen HD, Bashore TM et al, ACC/AHA Guidelines for cardiac catheterisation laboratories, *J Am Coll Cardiol* 1991; **18**: 1149–82.

5. Seldinger SI, Catheter replacement of the needle in percutaneous arteriography: a new technique, *Acta Radiol* 1953; **39**: 368–76.

6. Hildick-Smith DJR, Lowe MD, Walsh J et al, Coronary angiography from the radical artery: experience, complications and limitations, *Int J Cardiol* 1998; **64**: 231–9.

7. Sones FM Jr, Shirey EK, Proudfit WL et al, Cine-coronary arteriography, *Circulation* 1959; **20**: 773–4.

8. Webster JS, Moberg C, Rincon G, Natural history of severe proximal coronary artery disease as documented by coronary cineangiography, *Am J Cardiol* 1974; **33**: 195–200.

9. Harris PJ, Harrel FE, Lee KL et al, Survival in medically treated coronary artery disease, *Circulation* 1979; **60**: 1259–69.

10. Gould KL, Lipscomb K, Hamilton GW, Physiological basis for assessing critical coronary artery stenosis. Instantaneous flow response and regional distribution during coronary hyperaemia as measures of coronary flow reserve, *Am J Cardiol* 1974; **33**: 87–94.

11. Johnson LW, Lozner EC, Johnson S et al, Coronary arteriography 1984–1978: a report of the Society of Angiography and Interventions. Part I: results and complications, *Cathet Cardiovasc Diagn* 1989; **17**: 5–10.

12. Skillman JJ, Kim D, Bain DS, Vascular complications of percutaneous femoral cardiac interventions: incidence and operative repair, *Arch Surg* 1988; **123**: 1207–12.

13. Epstein AE, Davis KB, Kay GN et al, Significance of ventricular tachyarrythmias complicating cardiac catheterization: a CASS Registry study, *Am Heart J* 1990; **119**: 494–502.

14. Kennedy JW, Complications associated with cardiac catheterization and angiography, *Cathet Cardiovasc Diagn* 1982; **8**: 5–11.

Coronary angioplasty and stenting

Leonard M Shapiro

6

Interventional cardiology may be defined as the application of techniques based on cardiac catheterization to the treatment of coronary artery, valvular and congenital heart disease. Dotter and Judkins first performed a transluminal angioplasty to femoral artery stenosis in 1964.[1] Grüntzig introduced balloon dilatation of coronary arteries by modification and miniaturization of their technique. This was first performed in 1977 in Zurich,[2] where proximal left anterior descending coronary stenosis of a 37-year-old man was successfully dilated. The initial cases of balloon angioplasty were performed in young patients with stable symptoms, normal left ventricular contraction, and proximal well-localized stenoses, without visible radiological calcification in single coronary arteries. In the past few years, angioplasty has become much more widely used in many patients with stable angina, unstable coronary syndromes, and acute myocardial infarction. Coronary lesions that were previously unsuitable for dilatation, in that they were calcified, eccentric, distal occlusions, tortuous vessels, and in high-risk patients, are all now regularly performed.

From its early development, there has been a rapid growth in the number of interventional procedures performed. In Europe and the USA there has been a doubling of angioplasty procedures in the last 5 years and, in 1995, almost 900 000 cases were performed. Coincidentally, with the rapid growth in numbers of procedures performed, there have been technical developments of the equipment and imaging techniques. Until the early 1990s the vast majority of procedures were carried out by balloon dilatation alone. In the latter part of the 1990s there has been rapid development of a variety of new devices. Pre-eminent of these are intracoronary stents that provide a metal prosthetic scaffold. In addition, directional and rotational atherectomy to remove part of the bulk of a plaque, and laser procedures for recanalization, have also been used.

Equipment and procedure

The basic principles of coronary angioplasty have not changed since the first procedures undertaken by Grüntzig.[2] The procedures are carried out under local anaesthetic, possibly with a degree of systemic sedation. The coronary vessel is intubated by a guide catheter. This is a large lumen, thin-walled angiographic catheter, introduced from the femoral artery, or less commonly brachial or radial artery. High-quality radiographic images are obtained by contrast injections.

The projection(s) that best show the lesion to be dilated are usually frozen in the radiographic system and used as 'road maps' for the subsequent procedure. From such angiographic imaging, the type or nature of atherosclerotic lesion can be obtained. The American College of Cardiology classification into types A, B and C is a useful clinical guide to the subsequent success of the procedure. Type A are discrete accessible concentric lesions which have a high success rate at low risk. In comparison, type C have a lower success rate and higher risk. This includes diffuse or occluded lesions in tortuous vessels, with unprotected side-branches (Fig. 6.1). The distal end of the guiding catheter is coupled to a haemostatic seal with a side-port for contrast injection and pressure monitoring. Through this seal a guidewire is introduced into the coronary circulation. This is usually of diameter of 0.014 inch and is a type of construction which allows the transmission of torque from the external end. With a small angulation of the distal tip of the wire, this may be steered through stenoses and occlusions into the distal coronary circulation. Over this guiding wire is passed an angioplasty balloon. The evolution of the angioplasty balloon has been quite remarkable with progressive reduction in the deflated profiles so as to make crossing severe coronary occlusions or stenoses more easy to perform. The trackability and transmission of 'push' has also been improved. There are a variety of

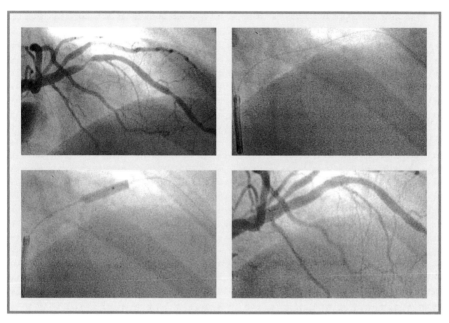

Figure 6.1
Coronary angioplasty. Severe proximal left anterior descending coronary artery lesion wire passage, balloon inflation, good angiographic outcome with a minimal residual stenosis.

types of shaft design and these also have to allow for the transmission of the inflating pressure. The common length for balloons is 2 cm, though a variety of other lengths are available for more specialized purposes. Once the balloon is passed across the stenotic or occluded area, it is inflated with diluted contrast so as to be visible by radiographic imaging. The balloon would be inflated to a preset diameter for relief of the vessel obstruction. Angina is a common but not invariable consequence of balloon dilatation and is relieved promptly by deflation of the balloon. A number of inflations, different dilatation pressures, and possibly balloon sizes, may be required for adequate relief of obstruction. Once this is complete and the angiographic result is satisfactory, other

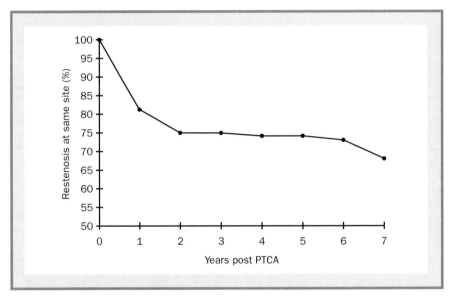

Figure 6.2
Restenosis rate following balloon angioplasty (Grüntzig 1978).

lesions in the same vessel or alternative parts of the coronary circulation can be dilated. Prior to an angioplasty procedure, patients would usually be pre-dosed with aspirin, and a systemic dose of heparin is given during the procedure.

There are many post-procedural regimens. It is usual for patients to be monitored 12–24 h for the development of recurrent myocardial ischaemia or haemorrhagic complications. The arterial sheaths are usually removed by direct pressure when the systemic heparinization has reversed. A variety of other methods and techniques are available for haemostasis.

Long-term outcome

Following a successful coronary angioplasty, the major factor which affects long-term event-free survival is restenosis (Fig. 6.2). There are a variety of definitions of restenosis, but the one most commonly used is a recurrence of a 50% narrowing at the site of the previous procedure.[3,4] Restenosis occurs in

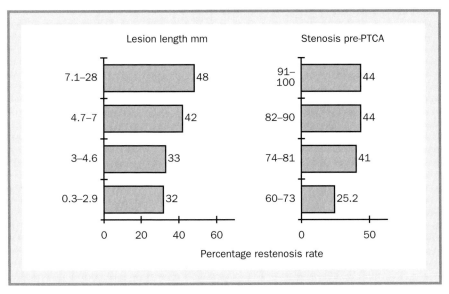

Figure 6.3
Factors influencing restenosis following balloon angioplasty (adapted from Hirshfeld et al 1991).

at least one-third of stenotic vessels and in up to 60% of those in whom dilatation has been performed in an occluded vessel or degenerate vein graft (Fig. 6.3). The majority of the restenosis occurs within 6 months of the procedure and the bulk of this within the first 3 months.[2] Early studies suggest that intimal proliferation was the major cause of arterial narrowing following injury. Multiple attempts at blocking intimal proliferation using a variety of agents have not shown any beneficial effects at present. More recent studies have suggested that there is little evidence of cellular proliferation in the 6-month period following angioplasty. Serial intravascular ultrasound shows that intimal thickening accounts for only a third of the loss of luminal diameter during this period. The majority of the loss of luminal diameter is made up by shrinkage or contraction of the dilated segment.

Angioplasty is one of the few technically complex and expensive procedures introduced

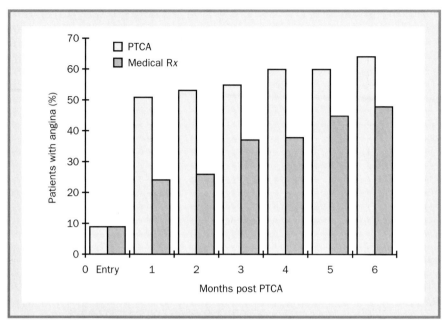

Figure 6.4
Comparison of PTCA and medical therapy for angina (adapted from Parisi et al 1992).

in modern times without extensive testing. Subsequent studies, however, have shown its benefits and limitations. Compared with medical therapy in patients with stable angina and single-vessel disease, it has been shown that angioplasty provides more complete relief of angina but with a higher rate for the need for further procedures (Fig. 6.4).[3] When comparing angioplasty to surgery, there are always higher rates of intervention in the former group. This relates to the risk of restenosis. The comparison studies including BARI and RITA show similar relief of angina in the long term, but the surgery group had a reduced need for further interventions. Even in single-vessel disease, there is a reduced risk of re-intervention in surgically treated groups. However, this is, of course, at the expense of a longer recovery period (Fig. 6.5).[5,7]

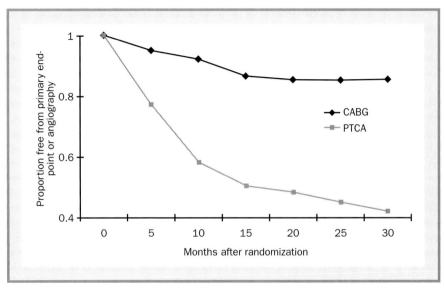

Figure 6.5
Comparison of PTCA versus bypass surgery for isolated proximal left artery descending disease.

Pathophysiology

The mechanism by which balloon angioplasty improves the size of the arterial lumen has been studied extensively in animal models, cadavers and specimens obtained from patients who died following successful or failed angioplasty procedures. More recently, the development of intracoronary ultrasound imaging has provided an additional and powerful method of studying the in vivo arterial response during and after angioplasty.

Balloon dilatation within a coronary artery leads to a radial force being exerted. This produces endothelial denudation with varying amounts of separation and fracture of the plaque from the underlying media. There may be stretching of the adventitial and medial layers and fracture and dissection of the media. Consequently, there are a number of mechanisms by which arterial dilatation may be achieved by balloon angioplasty. Although it was thought that plaque compression was important in the relief of obstruction, this probably only plays a minor role in the majority of patients with dense, fibrotic, and calcified stenoses. Balloon angioplasty largely acts by plaque fracture with the immediate formation of multiple fissures within the atherosclerotic plaque which allows channels for bloodflow. The subsequent outcome of the procedure in the short and long term is influenced by plaque healing and remodelling. Plaque fissuring, and medial and adventitial stretching, are seen in the post-angioplasty angiographic findings of intraluminal haziness in the area of localized vessel dilatation, in the presence of a discrete intimal flap or dissection. With the development of intracoronary ultrasound imaging, which allows high-quality views in the early post-PTCA situation, it is clear that there is extensive dissection of the arterial wall in more than 50% of patients. In the weeks following successful PTCA, favourable remodelling of the disrupted plaque and endothelialization of the areas of intimal injury usually result in increasing luminal size.

Because of the nature of vessel enlargement in balloon angioplasty, the single most important complication of this procedure is abrupt vessel closure. This occurs in 4–8% of cases, with the majority occurring while the patient is still in the cardiac catheterization laboratory. The mechanisms of abrupt coronary occlusion are similar to those noted from the procedure of balloon dilatation. Extensive dissection of the

medial layers can occur with obstructive dissection flaps or intramural haematoma. Exposure of subendothelial vascular wall results in platelet form deposition and activation and thrombotic occlusion.

The initial treatment for abrupt closure included prolonged balloon dilatation, often with a perfusion device. However, urgent surgery was often required, which frequently carried a high mortality and morbidity. Subsequent stent deployment effectively seals the dissection and restores normal flow.

Stent implantation

Although there have been many technological developments since the introduction of balloon angioplasty, intracoronary stenting may well be currently the most important.[8,9] Initial attempts were made to remove atherosclerotic plaque material by a variety of devices. This included directional atherectomy using a side-cutting device. Rotational devices are also available for pulverizing the plaque. Unfortunately, although these devices have a role in selected cases, they carry increased procedural risk and do not reduce the rate of restenosis. Therefore, stent implantation may be seen as an opportunity to avoid removal of plaque material but to scaffold or support the dilated area of artery. This has the advantage of eliminating acute and subacute elastic recoil, buttressing disrupted or friable

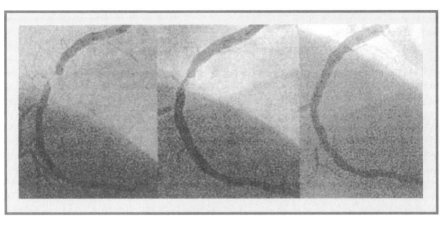

Figure 6.6
Stent into inadequate balloon dilation of right coronary artery.

atherosclerotic plaque material, and minimizing or reducing the contact between blood and injured subintimal arterial wall. In addition, the introduction of a stent allows an optimal dilatation of the vessel, achieving a larger final minimal luminal diameter. The initial applications of coronary stenting were for reducing the immediate need for bypass surgery for abrupt vessel closure.[5] As the problem is one of mechanical disruption, support of the ruptured segment, such as vessel dissection or plaque exclusion, leads to an excellent outcome (Fig. 6.6).

All dilated coronary arteries will renarrow, but the highest rate of restenosis is seen within degenerative vein grafts.[2] Balloon dilatation of such lesions is often very unsatisfactory, with acute closure of the vessel being a significant risk. In addition, the restenosis exceeds 75% in most circumstances. Implantation of stents of a variety of types greatly reduces the restenosis rate and makes the procedure safer in that it covers a large proportion of the friable atherosclerotic material within the vein graft and reduces the risk of acute closure and distal embolization. Recent trials in native coronary arteries, including BENE STENT and STRESS, have shown that there is a significant reduction in the rate of restenosis in patients undergoing stent implantation. It may be argued that the patients selected for randomized clinical trials comparing balloon angioplasty and stent implantation are a relatively small proportion of those undergoing clinical procedures. However, in these two studies, there was a substantial reduction in the number of patients who needed to undergo a repeat cardiac procedure or had any clinical endpoint (need for revascularization or myocardial infarction). The reduction of restenosis is seen very clearly in patients who have undergone recanalization of totally occluded vessels. The restenosis rate in such patients is particularly high and stent implantation gives a major reduction in the rate of restenosis. The implantation of an intracoronary stent probably prevents restenosis by its influence on the process of arterial remodelling. This is a process that has either an adaptive increase or pathological shrinkage in the sectional area of the artery. The process of adaptive remodelling has been well demonstrated to be present in non-dilated vessels, which delays the development of obstructive stenosis by progressive enlargement of the vessel in dilated vessels which do not stenose; such a process presumably occurs. Pathological remodelling allows the progressive encroachment of atheroma and neo-intima into the arterial lumen.[11–13]

Coronary stenting therefore reduces the rate of restenosis because it produces a large internal lumen. A larger lumen prevents early and late elastic recoil and alters the process of remodelling. Neo-intimal proliferation through the struts of the stent accounts for most of the late loss in arterial lumen, and there is little or no contribution from vessel shrinkage or modification of the cross-sectional area of the stent.

Subacute occlusion of coronary stents

Initial studies with stent implantation suggested that up to 10% of vessels would occlude abruptly in the 2-week period following the procedure. Initial attempts were made to prevent stent occlusion by intensive anticoagulant regimens. Following the procedure, aspirin, dipyridamole, dextran, heparin and warfarin have been given. This led to quite extensive bleeding complications and prolonged hospital stay. Intravascular ultrasound showed that Palmar–Schatz stents needed to be deployed at high inflation pressures so that the struts of the device were firmly opposed to the arterial wall brackets. With the development of stents which require lower inflation pressures and a clearer understanding of the need for full deployment, the risk of thrombotic complications has reduced to a very small value. The anti-coagulation regimen has now become concentrated on antiplatelet agents alone. Progressive developments in the design of stents is rapidly ongoing and current designs have considered adding anti-thrombotic agents such as heparin or other drugs to the design of the stent.

In-stent restenosis

While stent implantation yields larger minimal luminal diameter and beneficially modifies the process of arterial modelling, up to 10–20% of vessels will renarrow. The management of such restenoses remains unclear. Balloon dilatation will reduce the obstruction but at the expense of a high restenosis rate.[10] Rotational and directional atherectomy have limited application, and restenting may also be of benefit. Current research suggests that radiation therapy within the stent may reduce restenosis.

Conclusion

Coronary angioplasty has been a major technical advance in the management of patients with ischaemic heart disease. It relieves angina in patients with stenotic lesions. The development of coronary stent implantation has led to major advances in the practice of interventional cardiology, particularly by

preventing acute complication such as abrupt vessel closure and by reducing the rate of restenosis. Ongoing technical advances in stent design coatings and anti-thrombotic regimens will improve future procedures.

References

1. Dotter CT, Judkins MP, Transluminal treatment of arteriosclerotic obstruction. Description of a new technic and a preliminary report of its application, *Radiology* 1964; 172: 904–20.

2. Grüntzig A, Transluminal dilatation of coronary-artery stenosis, *Lancet* 1978; 1(8058): 263.

3. Hirshfeld JW Jr, Schwartz JS, Jugo R et al, Restenosis after coronary angioplasty: a multivariate statistical model to relate lesion and procedure variables to restenosis. The M-HEART Investigators, *J Am Coll Cardiol* 1991; 18: 647–56.

4. Savage MP, Goldberg S, Hirshfeld JW et al, Clinical and angiographic determinants of primary coronary angioplasty success. M-HEART, *J Am Coll Cardiol* 1991; 17(1): 22–8.

5. Parisi AF, Folland ED, Hartigan P, A comparison of angioplasty with medical therapy in the treatment of single-vessel coronary artery disease. Veterans Affairs ACME Investigators, *N Engl J Med* 1992; 326(1): 10–16.

6. Goy JJ, Eeckhout E, Burnand B et al, Coronary angioplasty versus left internal mammary artery grafting for isolated proximal left anterior descending artery stenosis, *Lancet* 1994; 343(8911): 1449–53.

7. Pocock SJ, Henderson RA, Rickards AF et al, Meta-analysis of randomised trials comparing coronary angioplasty with bypass surgery, *Lancet* 1995; **346**(8984): 1184–9.

8. Goy JJ, Eeckhout E, Intracoronary stenting, *Lancet* 1998; **351**(9120): 1943–9.

9. Ellis SG, Savage M, Fischman D et al, Restenosis after placement of Palmaz–Schatz stents in native coronary arteries. Initial results of a multicenter experience, *Circulation* 1992; **86**(6): 1836–44.

10. Macaya C, Serruys PW, Ruygrok P et al, Continued benefit of coronary stenting versus balloon angioplasty: one-year clinical follow-up of Benestent trial. Benestent Study Group, *J Am Coll Cardiol* 1996; **27**(2): 255–61.

11. Serruys PW, van Hout B, Bonnier H et al, Randomised comparison of implantation of heparin-coated stents with balloon angioplasty in selected patients with coronary artery disease (Benestent II), *Lancet* 1998; **352**(9129): 673–81.

12. Laham RJ, Carrozza JP, Berger C et al, Long-term (4- to 6-year) outcome of Palmaz–Schatz stenting: paucity of late clinical stent-related problems, *J Am Coll Cardiol* 1996; **28**(4): 820–6.

13. Serruys PW, Emanuelsson H, van der Giessen W et al, Heparin-coated Palmaz–Schatz stents in human coronary arteries. Early outcome of the Benestent-II, *Circulation* 1996; **93**(3): 412–22.

Management of arrhythmias associated with coronary artery disease

Yee Guan Yap and Edward Rowland

7

Introduction

Despite the tremendous strides in management over recent years, coronary heart disease remains the leading cause of death in the industrialized world. In the UK it is estimated that the incidence of sudden death is in the region of 1500 per million population, and this represents only a small proportion of those dying as a consequence of coronary disease.[1] Most deaths following an acute myocardial infarction (AMI) occur in the first year, with mortality rates ranging from 5% to 15%.[2,3] The major cause of death in the first year after AMI is sudden death, usually due to ventricular arrhythmia.[4,5] While the mechanism and even the definition of sudden death is still much debated,[6] it is recognized that the majority of these events, although not exclusively, begin as ventricular tachycardia which degenerates into ventricular fibrillation and occurs in the absence of either acute infarction or significant ischaemia.[7,8]

When a coronary artery is occluded or narrowed, the electrical function of the myocardium or conduction system subtended may be altered or destroyed. This may lead to disorders of impulse formation of conduction and can be expressed in many different rhythm abnormalities. They may occur in the setting of AMI, can occur (often years) after infarction and can complicate myocardial ischaemia in coronary artery disease (CAD) without previous infarction. In addition to the ventricular arrhythmias, other important electrical complications include atrial fibrillation (AF), sinus node dysfunction, and AV block. AF can present as a complication of myocardial ischaemia or can be a pre-existing condition. In a database of more than 40 000 patients with AMI treated with thrombolytic therapy, 2.5% of the patients had pre-existing AF on admission, and a further 7.9% of patients developed AF during hospitalization.[9] Heart block of various forms can occur in the context of myocardial infarction or may develop during follow-up. It can have important therapeutic and prognostic implications[10] but has not been the focus of major new developments and will not be covered in this chapter.

Arrhythmias remain a major complication in patients with CAD and an important public health issue. The management of atrial fibrillation and flutter, ventricular tachycardia and sudden death associated with CAD will be discussed in this chapter.

Atrial fibrillation

AF can cause distressing symptoms such as palpitation and shortness of breath, or may be asymptomatic. It can precipitate ischaemic syndromes and heart failure. AF is also associated with up to twice the risk for total mortality and cardiovascular death,[11,12] while the risk of stroke can be increased fivefold with AF.[13] As in other patient populations, the stroke risk can be alleviated by appropriate anticoagulant treatment — there is as yet little evidence that the non-embolic risk can be attenuated by anti-arrhythmic therapy.

AF is classified into paroxysmal, persistent or permanent forms[14] (Table 7.1). While such a

Table 7.1
Classification of atrial fibrillation and treatment strategies

Type	Duration and character
Paroxysmal	<2–7 days, frequently <24 h. Spontaneous conversion occurs frequently
Persistent	>2–7 days. Usually electrical cardioversion needed to restore sinus rhythm
Permanent	Restoration of sinus rhythm not feasible

classification is based on the temporal pattern of the condition and does not reflect the underlying pathophysiological mechanism, it helps in the planning of treatment strategies for the condition. Before treating a patient with AF, it is necessary to consider the patient's symptomatology and the prognostic implications if the arrhythmia is allowed to persist or recur. The treatment strategy for AF is dependent on the therapeutic end-points. Essentially, the treatment of AF can be broadly divided into three strategies:[15]

1. Restoration of sinus rhythm with electrical or pharmacological cardioversion.
2. Maintenance of sinus rhythm in paroxysmal AF and persistent AF after cardioversion.
3. Control of the ventricular rate during a paroxysm of AF or during the presence of persistent or permanent AF.

Restoration of sinus rhythm

All patients with persistent AF should be considered for cardioversion by drugs or direct current (DC) shock regardless of symptoms unless there are contraindications to cardioversion. Cardioversion is only worthwhile if it is the first presentation with persistent AF or when, following relapse, appropriate efforts are going to be made to maintain sinus rhythm after cardioversion.

Each patient will require individual assessment of the probability of successful cardioversion and the likelihood of maintaining sinus rhythm thereafter (Table 7.2). Several factors have been shown to correlate with the outcome of cardioversion and recurrence of AF. Patients age >50 years and with underlying rheumatic mitral valve disease are associated with a poor success rate of cardioversion,[16,17] whereas prolonged duration of AF (>1 year), large atrial size (>55 mm), rheumatic mitral valve disease and low functional class (≥NYHA III)[18–20] are associated with recurrence of AF. These factors are derived from DC cardioversion but the same factors are probably relevant for pharmacological cardioversion. It is also clear that AF has a higher recurrence rate when it occurs in the acute phase of myocardial infarction and after cardiac surgery — it is often more prudent to await the passage of time, if necessary controlling an excessive ventricular rate, until the calmer circumstances of the subacute phase.

For acute pharmacological cardioversion, class Ic drugs are the most effective compared to class III agents.[21] However, following the CAST study,[22] where flecainide demonstrated an increased mortality when given to post-myocardial infarction patients, they are probably best avoided in all patients with CAD. Although subgroup analysis identified particular patient characteristics which placed

Table 7.2
Indications and contraindications for cardioversion.

Indications
  Recent onset of atrial fibrillations, even if asymptomatic
  History of peripheral embolic episodes
  Persistent AF
  Rapid ventricular rate unresponsive to medical therapy
  Persistent symptoms on medical therapy
Contraindications
  Relative
    Atrial fibrillation >2 years
    Left atrial dimension >50 mm
    NYHA class III or IV
    LVEF <25%
  Absolute
    Digitalis toxicity
    Patients with sinus node dysfunction and tachybrady syndrome, unless a
      pacemaker is implanted

the subject at risk of the pro-arrhythmic complications, caution would seem to be appropriate at present. Intravenous amiodarone is not effective for acute conversion (<1 h) but may still be useful for late conversion and is successful in over 80% of patients within 24 h.[15] Oral amiodarone can also be used to restore sinus rhythm in patients with persistent AF (>3 weeks) but is only successful in 50% of patients.[15]

In patients with persistent AF following acute myocardial infarction, the choice of treatment is between intravenous amiodarone and DC cardioversion. Intravenous amiodarone is preferred in stable patients, whereas DC cardioversion is mandatory whenever the arrhythmia precipitates heart failure or severe angina.[21]

DC cardioversion will convert approximately 90% of patients with chronic AF.[23] All patients undergoing electrical cardioversion will require oral anticoagulation for 3 weeks prior to the procedure and for 4 weeks afterwards.[24–26] In recent-onset AF, it is generally thought to be safe to cardiovert without anticoagulation if cardioversion is undertaken within 48 h.[15] However, in practice, intravenous heparin should be given upon diagnosis while the decision on the appropriateness of DC cardioversion and the preparation for the procedure is carried out. This should then be followed by 4 weeks of warfarin therapy. If there is left atrial dilatation and/or mitral valve disease, formal oral anticoagulant treatment for 3 weeks is preferable prior to DC cardioversion, even if the onset is within 48 h.

Hypokalaemia and supratherapeutic levels of digoxin can precipitate ventricular arrhythmias with DC cardioversion — if serum potassium is normal, the risk of ventricular arrhythmias is so low that checking digoxin levels is generally unnecessary. Cardioversion should be undertaken with an initial 200- or 300-J shock. A maximum of two further 360-J shocks can be tried. Cardioversion should be abandoned if it is unsuccessful after the third shock. A further cardioversion attempt should be made after 6 weeks of treatment with amiodarone. Both amiodarone and esmolol have been shown to improve the probability of successful cardioversion, or the maintenance of sinus rhythm after successful cardioversion.[27,28] After successful DC cardioversion, it may take at least 3 weeks for full atrial mechanical activity to restore.[29] It is therefore important that both the anti-arrhythmic and anticoagulant therapy is continued at least until this period.

Maintenance of sinus rhythm

The maintenance of sinus rhythm is an important treatment strategy in patients with paroxysmal AF or persistent AF. Class Ic anti-arrhythmic drugs are effective for this purpose but are contraindicated in patients after myocardial infarction for reasons given above. Common sense dictates that their harmful effects will also be seen in those with CAD and no previous infarction — therefore, their use should be avoided in all CAD patients. The class 1a group of anti-arrhythmic drugs, such as procainamide and disopyramide, has not been evaluated extensively and the studies available are limited. They have fallen out of vogue because of the pro-arrhythmic risk (quinidine) or because of side-effects and tendency to aggravate left ventricular dyfunction (disopyramide). Beta-blockers offer an alternative, although one which, with the exception of sotalol, does not provide an especially high efficacy rate. Sotalol has shown equivalent efficacy rates to quinidine in the prevention of AF[30] but is ineffective for acute conversion.

Amiodarone is effective in maintaining sinus rhythm in 53–97% of patients with chronic AF or paroxysmal AF and is especially useful in patients refractory to other drugs.[31–36] In contrast to class Ic drugs, amiodarone is rarely pro-arrhythmic and is particularly useful in patients after acute myocardial infarction with or with left ventricular dysfunction.[37] However, the relatively high incidence of side-effects of amiodarone[36,37] limits its long-term value and will increase the attractiveness of alternative non-pharmacological strategies.

Newer anti-arrhythmic drugs and anti-arrhythmic therapies

The data on newer class III anti-arrhythmics such as ibutilide and dofetilide are currently undergoing clinical evaluation. The use of dofetilide for the reduction of mortality in patients with left ventricular dysfunction after myocardial infarction has been investigated in the two Danish Investigation of Arrhythmias and Mortality on Dofetilide (DIAMOND) trials.[38] One trial enrolled patients within 7 days of an acute myocardial infarction (DIAMOND-MI), while the other randomized patients with acute congestive heart failure (DIAMOND-CHF). The preliminary results of both trials showed that dofetilide has a neutral effect on total mortality, a relatively low incidence of torsade de pointes and a beneficial effect in reducing the development of AF in those who started the trial in sinus rhythm. Dofetilide was also effective in converting to sinus rhythm and maintaining in sinus rhythm those initially in AF.[39] Thus, dofetilide appears to be safe in patients with ischaemic heart disease.

The last decade has seen an explosion in the development of non-pharmacological therapies for the treatment of cardiac arrhythmias. AF may be prevented by 'maze' surgery, which prevents the occurrence of AF by placement of multiple atrial incisions. Catheter-based operations to reproduce these results are in their infancy but will become a reality. At present, direct atrial ablation for AF is restricted to those who have the 'focal' form. An implantable atrial defibrillator capable of delivering low-energy DC shocks to the atrium offers a further novel method of treatment for the resistant case.

Control of ventricular rate

AF may result in an uncontrolled ventricular rate and this may lead to symptoms or haemodynamic compromise. Control of the ventricular rate is valuable in the following situations:

- when there is a relapse in patients with paroxysmal AF
- when AF occurs acutely and cardioversion cannot be undertaken promptly
- in permanent AF.

Adequate rate control has the potential to improve quality of life, alleviate distressing symptoms and prevent or reverse left ventricular dysfunction. Generally, a target resting heart rate of below 90 beats/min at rest and below 110 beats/min during light and moderate exercise should be the aim.[15] There are three classes of drugs to choose from for rate control: digoxin, beta-blockers and calcium channel blockers. The American Heart Association suggests that verapamil should be used in most patients, whereas the Canadian College of Cardiology suggests digoxin as the drug of choice.[40,41] Digoxin provides rate control at rest but its effect is not maintained during exercise — it is therefore useful in the elderly, whose levels of activity may be modest. The dose should be titrated against resting heart rate.[15] On the other hand, beta-blockers, diltiazem and verapamil may reduce peak heart rate excessively and limit the exercise tolerability. They will therefore need to be titrated to provide control of both resting and daily exercise heart rate.[15] Both should be used cautiously for fear of aggravating unsuspected heart failure due to their negative inotropic effects — beta-blockers may be preferred in the context of coronary heart disease.

Atrial flutter

This arrhythmia is important to distinguish from AF. Not only does it have important distinguishing clinical features, but there are important therapeutic differences. Atrial flutter is not unusual in patients with CAD and particularly after coronary artery bypass grafting. The ventricular response in atrial flutter tends to be higher than in AF. There is a risk of 1 : 1 AV conduction, and any anti-arrhythmic drug that acts at the atrial level (classes 1 and III) should be co-administered with a drug that slows AV conduction to protect against this possibility. In general, atrial flutter tends to be more difficult to prevent with anti-arrhythmic drugs than AF. AF and atrial flutter often co-exist, in the same patient, and it is not unusual to be able to control the former but not the latter.

Atrial flutter in its classical form depends upon a re-entrant wavefront of excitation that must pass through the narrow isthmus between the tricuspid annulus and the inferior vena cava (IVC). Recently, it has been possible to create an ablation line across this isthmus — if conduction via the isthmus is prevented, atrial flutter cannot occur.[42]

Anticoagulant therapy

Aspirin will nowadays be in routine use in those with CAD, irrespective of whether they have AF. In general, aspirin is used as adequate protection against thromboembolic events in those who are at low risk, that is young patients (<65 years of age) who are free of history of hypertension, cerebral vascular disease, congestive heart failure or diabetes,[43] or in patients for whom warfarin is contraindicated. Oral anticoagulant should be considered in patients with frequent episodes of uncontrolled AF, in patients requiring DC cardioversion (see above), and in the long-term management of permanent AF. For non-rheumatic AF, the annual risk of ischaemic stroke is 4.5%, reduced to 1.4% per year with warfarin, and there is an overall relative risk reduction of 68%.[44] While the risk of major haemorrhage, including cerebral haemorrhage, is 1.3% per year with warfarin compared with 1% in the controls,[44] warfarin still confers an overall benefit (in those <75 years of age). Aspirin has a lower risk of major haemorrhage but only reduces the risk of ischaemic stroke by 21%.[44] Generally, an International Normalized Ratio (INR) range of 2.0–3.0 with a target of 2.5 is optimal for the majority of patients.[43] However, in patients with previous transient ischaemic attacks or minor stroke, a higher range of 2.0–3.9 with a target of 3.0 should be the aim — in those patients with higher risk of cerebral haemorrhage, a range of 1.6–2.5 with a target of 2.0 is sufficient.[43]

Ventricular arrhythmias

Ventricular arrhythmias (ventricular tachycardia and ventricular fibrillation) are life-threatening complications after myocardial infarction. Myocardial ischaemia and infarction provide an electrophysiological milieu favourable for the initiation and maintenance of ventricular tachyarrhythmia. Different electrophysiological mechanisms are involved in the genesis of ventricular arrhythmias at different stages after myocardial infarction. In the early stages of AMI, ventricular arrhythmia is attributed to re-entry, whereas at 6–8 h the mechanism of ventricular arrhythmia is due to abnormal automaticity.[45] Late arrhythmia, however, is again attributed to a re-entrant mechanism. Ventricular fibrillation occurs most frequently in the earliest minutes of AMI, and declines exponentially thereafter.[46] Ventricular fibrillation complicates about 5% of patients hospitalized for AMI.[47] Ventricular tachycardia occurs in up to 67% of patients in the acute phase of myocardial infarction but most of these events are short-lived — although they may have some immediate haemodynamic effect, they are usually asymptomatic because of their brevity.[48] The important and distinctive feature of an early ventricular arrhythmia (within the first 24–36 h) is that it is a transient phase and, in the absence of severe left ventricular dysfunction, does not leave the patient necessarily prone to future arrhythmic events. Sustained monomorphic ventricular tachycardia is not a typical arrhythmia in the subacute phase of myocardial infarction.

The treatment strategy for ventricular arrhythmia should target the cause of the arrhythmia as well as the underlying pathophysiology. In other words, in patients with significant CAD, revascularization should be considered in the first instance and, if the patient has left ventricular dysfunction, effective treatment of heart failure pursued. It is only when these have been achieved or are inappropriate or unnecessary that direct anti-arrhythmic strategies should be employed. It is intriguing to speculate that the increased use of thrombolytic therapy has not only reduced the immediate mortality from acute myocardial syndromes but has also had an impact on the long-term arrhythmic burden.

Acute treatment of ventricular arrhythmias

Ventricular fibrillation and pulseless ventricular tachycardia cause instant circulatory collapse and cardiac arrest. Resuscitation with immediate cardioversion should be initiated following the UK Resuscitation Council guidelines (Fig. 7.1).

If sustained ventricular tachycardia is causing haemodynamic compromise, prompt treatment is necessary. Electrolyte imbalance can precipitate ventricular tachycardia and should be checked. Intravenous lignocaine is safe and effective and should be the first-line drug for acute termination of ventricular tachycardia. If ventricular tachycardia does not respond to lignocaine, intravenous amiodarone is a useful second-line drug[49] but may take up to 24 h to work. Cardioversion is needed if anti-arrhythmic drugs are

ineffective, are contraindicated or cause haemodynamic deterioration. Drugs such as flecainide and sotalol, when used orally, cause an increase in mortality associated with their use in post-myocardial infarction patients,[50,51] and there is no rationale for their intravenous use for the treatment of ventricular tachycardia. Other anti-arrhythmic drugs such as propafenone and disopyramide have been used for the acute treatment of ventricular tachycardia after acute myocardial infarction. Their adverse effects on left ventricular contractility and pro-arrhythmic potential[52–54] mean they should be used with extreme caution in these circumstances.

If drugs are ineffective, overdrive pacing may be used to terminate ventricular tachycardia and is especially valuable in the temporary management of recurrent, frequent or incessant ventricular tachycardia. Right ventricular burst pacing for 3–10 s at a rate 10–30% in excess of the tachycardia will often terminate the tachycardia.

Secondary prevention of ventricular arrhythmias

It has been clear that patients with CAD who present with sustained ventricular arrhythmia have a high rate of recurrent arrhythmia and a significant long term mortality. The lack of randomized studies has hindered the determination of the precise level of risk and

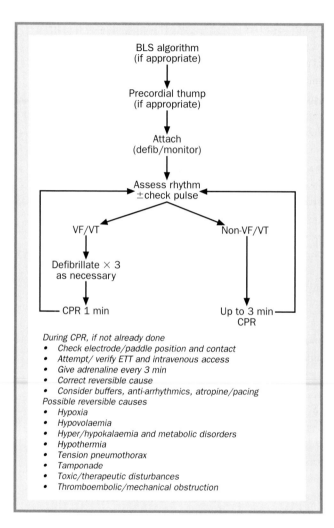

Figure 7.1
*Resuscitation algorithm
(Resuscitation Council UK
1997).*

BLS algorithm
(if appropriate)

Precordial thump
(if appropriate)

Attach
(defib/monitor)

Assess rhythm
±check pulse

VF/VT   Non-VF/VT

Defibrillate × 3
as necessary

CPR 1 min   Up to 3 min
                        CPR

During CPR, if not already done
- *Check electrode/paddle position and contact*
- *Attempt/ verify ETT and intravenous access*
- *Give adrenaline every 3 min*
- *Correct reversible cause*
- *Consider buffers, anti-arrhythmics, atropine/pacing*

Possible reversible causes
- *Hypoxia*
- *Hypovolaemia*
- *Hyper/hypokalaemia and metabolic disorders*
- *Hypothermia*
- *Tension pneumothorax*
- *Tamponade*
- *Toxic/therapeutic disturbances*
- *Thromboembolic/mechanical obstruction*

identification of precise risk factors. However, it is clear that the extent of left ventricular dysfunction, method of initial presentation (syncopal versus haemodynamic tolerance), number of previous infarcts, etc. are some of the factors that identify the higher-risk patient. Whether anti-arrhythmic drug therapy was able to improve the outcome in these patients was never established in a properly controlled fashion. The arrival of the implantable cardioverter–defibrillator (ICD), with its demonstrable ability to terminate spontaneous ventricular tachycardia or ventricular fibrillation, has clarified some, but certainly not all, of the uncertainty surrounding the value of therapeutic strategies in these populations.

The Antiarrhythmic Versus Implantable Defibrillator (AVID) study showed that the ICD reduced mortality compared with amiodarone or sotalol in patients with ventricular fibrillation or haemodynamically unstable or poorly tolerated ventricular tachycardia.[55] Although the study enrolled patients with all forms of heart disease, those with CAD were the majority — the benefit of ICD therapy was seen equally among those with dilated cardiomyopathy and those with coronary disease. At a follow-up of 18 months, the mortality rates were 15.8 ± 3.2% for the ICD compared with 24.4 ± 3.7% for drugs. The relative risk reductions at 1, 2 and 3 years were 39 ± 20%, 27 ± 21% and

31 ± 21%. However, the benefit of ICD therapy was only seen in those with an ejection fraction of 36% or less, and the averaged unadjusted lifetime extension conferred by ICD at 3 years was only 3.2 months. It may be argued that this latter figure underestimated the value of the therapy because the study was terminated prematurely when statistical analysis at an interim data point revealed the statistical superiority of the ICD limb. The only confounding discrepancy in the study was that a greater proportion of the ICD patients were taking beta-blockers than in the medically treated group (mostly amiodarone). The Canadian Implantable Defibrillator Study (CIDS) and Cardiac Arrest Study Hamburg (CASH) have also evaluated the treatment effect of ICD versus anti-arrhythmic drugs.[56,57] The trials are now complete and the preliminary results complement those of AVID.

The results of the AVID trial provide compelling evidence that the ICD is the preferred treatment in patients who have CAD, and an ejection fraction of 35% or below, and who present with ventricular fibrillation, ventricular tachycardia with syncope, or ventricular tachycardia accompanied by hypotension or chest pain, and where it is not associated with a transient or reversible cause.

Sudden cardiac death

Sudden cardiac death, largely resulting from ventricular arrhythmias, is a major cause of death in the first year after AMI.

The identification of patients at risk of developing life-threatening ventricular arrhythmias following AMI remains a healthcare priority. Several risk parameters, such as left ventricular ejection fraction, signal-averaged ECG and ventricular premature complexes, are limited in their usefulness due to low sensitivity and a high number of false-positive results. Recently, it has been shown that heart rate variability and baroreflex sensitivity have independent prognostic values in the prediction of cardiac death (sudden and non-sudden) for patients after myocardial infarction, particularly if both were depressed.[58] However, the positive predictive value remains low at 15% when both heart rate variability and baroreflex sensitivity were depressed. Furthermore, it is not yet certain whether high-risk patients selected by both depressed heart rate variability and depressed baroreflex sensitivity can benefit from either pharmacological or non-pharmacological therapies. Therefore, the selection of patients at risk of sudden death after myocardial infarction remains a challenge.

Recognition of the relatively high rate of arrhythmic death has prompted the search for an effective prophylactic anti-arrhythmic drug for the prevention of sudden cardiac death following an AMI. Apart from beta-blockers,[59–61] no other agent has been conclusively shown to reduce mortality. Indeed, several recent randomized clinical trials showed that some anti-arrhythmic agents increased the mortality. Both the CAST and SWORD studies demonstrated that the prophylactic use of class I agents (encanide, flecainide or moricizine) and the class III agent (d-sotalol) increased the mortality in postinfarction patients.[50,51,62] Amiodarone is an exception. It blocks multiple ion channels, has potent anti-arrhythmic effects and usually does not impair left ventricular function. Despite these favourable actions, two major postinfarction studies (EMIAT and CAMIAT), using either left ventricular dysfunction or ventricular premature depolarizations respectively as surrogate marker of high risk, failed to demonstrate any improvement in total mortality. Interestingly, while amiodarone reduced arrhythmic death in these high-risk post-myocardial infarction patients, the observation that there was no reduction in the total mortality between amiodarone and placebo groups suggests that a benefit on prevention of lethal arrhythmia was counteracted by an adverse outcome in those with ischaemic events.[63,64]

Ever since the early days of the ICD, it has been clear that it is effective for treating ventricular fibrillation and ventricular tachycardia. If anti-arrhythmic drug therapy is ineffective in preventing sudden death, an alternative strategy is to identify those patients who are at risk postinfarction and use the ICD to treat any potentially lethal ventricular arrhythmia. The MADIT and CABG-Patch trials evaluated the ability of ICD to reduce the risk of sudden death in coronary artery patients without previous life-threatening ventricular arrhythmias.[65,66] In the MADIT trial, 196 patients in NYHA functional class I–III with prior myocardial infarction were identified as high risk by at least one episode of documented asymptomatic non-sustained ventricular tachycardia on ECG monitoring, left ventricular ejection fraction of ≤35%, and inducible sustained ventricular tachycardia on electrophysiological study that was not suppressed with procainamide. The patients were then randomized to either ICD or conventional therapy (amiodarone in the majority of patients). The trial was terminated prematurely due to the marked reduction in all-cause mortality in the ICD group. At an average follow-up of 2.25 years, the hazard ratio was 0.46 (95% CI = 0.26–0.82, $p = 0.009$), indicating a reduction in mortality of more than 50% with ICD therapy. However, there were several problems with this trial. When the cause of death was examined, the ICD group had a reduction not only in arrhythmic death (13 versus 3), but also in non-arrhythmic cardiac death (13 versus 7) and death of unknown causes (6 versus 0),

unexplained discrepancies for which there is no plausible explanation. Furthermore, in the conventional therapy group, amiodarone was used in 74% of the patients 1 month after randomization and 45% at the time of last contact, and beta-blockers and angiotensin-converting enzyme inhibitors were used in only 5% and 51% of patients respectively. Finally, no registry was kept on the proportion, characteristics and outcome of patients who met the initial entry criteria but who had no inducible ventricular tachycardia on electrophysiological study. All of these problems make it difficult to assess the result of MADIT in clinical practice. Nevertheless, this is the first prospective randomized trial which demonstrates that prophylactic ICD therapy improved survival compared with conventional antiarrhythmic therapy.

The CABG-Patch trial[66] compared the impact of ICD with control on all-cause mortality in patients with ischaemic heart disease, left ventricular ejection fraction <36% and abnormal signal-averaged ECG undergoing coronary artery revascularization. A total of 900 patients were randomized (446 to ICD and 454 to control) and use of anti-arrhythmic drugs was similar between the two groups. During a follow-up of 32 ± 16 months, there were 101 deaths in the ICD group and 95 in the control group. The hazard ratio was 1.07 (95% CI = 0.81–1.42), indicating no benefit from ICD in this patient population.

The results of MADIT and CABG-Patch studies provide complementary evidence on the use of prophylactic ICD for the prevention of sudden cardiac death in high-risk patients with CAD. It is likely that the CABG-Patch trial did not select patients at high risk of arrhythmic death and/or that coronary artery bypass graft surgery reduced the risk of arrhythmic death to the degree that there were few deaths potentially prevented by ICD therapy.[67] Moreover, inducible sustained ventricular tachycardia on electrophysiological study, itself a powerful predictor of arrhythmic events, was not used to stratify patients in the CABG-Patch trial and may account for the difference in the hazard ratios in both trials. At present, there is not enough compelling evidence to support the prophylactic use of ICD in the prevention of sudden death in patients with CAD. The result of other ongoing studies such as the Multicenter Unsustained Tachycardia Trial (MUSST), which addresses the same population as MADIT but uses a different design and a control group which receives no anti-arrhythmic therapy, will help to clarify the roles of ICD in the prevention of sudden cardiac death.[68]

Conclusion

AF and ventricular arrhythmias remain the major complications in patients with CAD. At present, anti-arrhythmic drugs are the mainstays of treatment for AF. The advent of novel anti-arrhythmic techniques such as catheter ablation and the internal atrial defibrillator will change the treatment strategy for AF in the future.

While the ICD has provided promising results compared with anti-arrhythmic drug in the secondary prevention of patients with ventricular arrhythmias, its role in the primary prevention of sudden cardiac death remains undefined. It is important to appreciate that the identification of patients at risk of sudden cardiac death remains a challenge and will have an impact on the selection of patients for prophylactic treatment of sudden cardiac death.

References

1. Boaz A, Rayner M, Coronary Heart Disease Statistics, The Coronary Prevention Group/British Heart Foundation Statistics Database, 1995.

2. Frishman WH, Furberg CD, Friedewald WT, Beta-adrenergic blockade for survivors of acute myocardial infarction, *N Engl J Med* 1984; **310**: 830–7.

3. The Multicenter Postinfarction Research Group, Risk stratification and survival after myocardial infarction, *N Engl J Med* 1983; **309**: 331–6.

4. Rosenthal ME, Oseran DS, Gang E, Peter T, Sudden cardiac death following acute myocardial infarction, *Am Heart J* 1985; **109**: 865–75.

5. Bayes de Luna A, Coumel P, Leclercq JF, Ambulatory sudden cardiac death: mechanisms of production of fatal arrhythmia on the basis of data from 157 cases, *Am Heart J* 1989; **117:** 151–9.

6. Hinkle LE, Thaler HT, Clinical classification of cardiac deaths, *Circulation* 1982; **65:** 457–64.

7. Rapaport E, Sudden cardiac death, *Am J Cardiol* 1988; **62:** 31–61.

8. Kempf FC, Josephson ME, Cardiac arrest recorded on ambulatory electrocardiograms, *Am J Cardiol* 1984; **53:** 1577–82.

9. Grenshaw BS, Ward SR, Granger CB et al, Atrial fibrillation in the setting of acute myocardial infarction: the GUSTO–1 experience, *J Am Coll Cardiol* 1997; **30:** 406–13.

10. Goldberg RJ, Zevallos JC, Yarzebski J et al, Prognosis of acute myocardial infarction complicated by complete heart block (the Worcester Heart Attack Study), *Am J Cardiol* 1992; **69:** 1135–41.

11. Kannel WB, Abbott RD, Savage DD, McNamara PM, Epidemiologic features of atrial fibrillation: the Framingham study, *N Engl J Med* 1982; **306:** 1018–22.

12. Krahn DA, Manfreda J, Tate BR, Mathewson FAL, Cuddy TE, Prognosis of atrial fibrillation in men. Manitoba Follow-up Study (MFUS), *J Am Coll Cardiol* 1993; **21:** 478A.

13. Wolf PA, Abbot R, Kennel W, Atrial fibrillation as an independent risk factor for stroke: the Framingham study, *Stroke* 1991; **22:** 983–8.

14. Gallagher MM, Camm AJ, Classification of atrial fibrillation, *PACE* 1997; **20:** 1603–5.

15. Crijns HJGM, Van Gelder IC, Tieleman RG,

Van Gilst WH, Atrial fibrillation: antiarrhythmic therapy. In: Yusuf S, Cairns JA, Camm AJ, Fallen EL, Gersh BJ, eds, *Evidence based Cardiology* (BMJ Books: London, 1998) 527–43.

16. Brodsky MA, Allen BJ, Capparelli EV, Luckett CR, Morton R, Henry WL, Factors determining maintenance of sinus rhythm after cardioversion in chronic atrial fibrillation with left atrial dilatation, *Am J Cardiol* 1989; **63:** 1065–8.

17. Waris E, Kreus KE, Salokannel J, Factors influencing persistence of sinus rhythm after DC shock treatment of atrial fibrillation, *Acta Med Scand* 1971; **189:** 161–6.

18. Szekeley P, Sideris D, Batson G, Maintenance of sinus rhythm after atrial fibrillation, *Br Heart J* 1970; **32:** 741–6.

19. Van Gelder IC, Crijns HJGM, Tieleman RG et al, Value and limitation of electrical cardioversion in patients with chronic atrial fibrillation — importance of arrhythmia risk factors and oral anticoagulation, *Arch Intern Med* 1996; **156:** 2585–92.

20. Crijns HJGM, Gosselink ATM, Van Gelder IC et al, Drugs after cardioversion to prevent relapses of chronic atrial fibrillation. In: Kingma JH, van Hemel NM, Lie KI, eds, *Atrial Fibrillation, a Treatable Disease?* (Kluwer Academic Publishers: Dordrecht, 1992) 105–48.

21. Fresco C, Proclemer A, on behalf of the PAFIT-2 Investigators, Management of recent onset atrial fibrillation, *Eur Heart J* 1996; **17** (suppl C): C41–7.

22. The Cardiac Arrhythmia Suppression Trial Investigators, Preliminary reports: effect of encainide and flecainide on mortality in a randomised trial of arrhythmia suppression

after myocardial infarction, *N Engl J Med* 1989; **321**: 406–12.

23. Lown B, Amarasingham R, Neuman J, New method for terminating cardiac arrhythmias, *JAMA* 1962; **182**: 548–55.

24. Laupacis A, Albers G, Dalend et al, Antithrombotic therapy in atrial fibrillation, *Chest* 1995; **108**: 352S–95.

25. Manning WJ, Leeman DE, Gotch PJ et al, Pulsed Doppler evaluation of atrial mechanical function after electrical cardioversion of atrial fibrillation, *J Am Coll Cardiol* 1989; **13**: 617–23.

26. Padraig GO, Puleo PR, Bolli R et al, Return of atrial mechanical function following electrical cardioversion of atrial dysrhythmia, *Am Heart J* 1990; **120**: 353–9.

27. Newby KH, Waugh R, Hardee M, Henderson PH, Mertz J, Natale A, Amiodarone decreases defibrillation threshold in patients undergoing elective cardioversion for atrial fibrillation, *Circulation* 1996; **94**: I-667.

28. Niebauer M, Chung MK, Holmes D, Van Wagoner DR, Tchou P, Esmolol reduces atrial defibrillation thresholds: a randomised, placebo-controlled study, *J Am Coll Cardiol* 1997; **29**: 292A.

29. Manning WJ, Leeman DE, Gotch PJ, Come PC, Pulsed Doppler evaluation of atrial mechanical function after electrical cardioversion of atrial fibrillation, *J Am Coll Cardiol* 1989; **13**: 617–23.

30. Juul-Moller S, Edvardsson N, Rehnquist-Ahlberg N, Sotalol versus quinidine for the maintenance of sinus rhythm after direct-current cardioversion of atrial fibrillation, *Circulation* 1990; **82**: 1932–9.

31. Vitolo E, Tronci M, Larovere MT, Rumolo R, Morabito A, Amiodarone versus quinidine in the prophylaxis of atrial fibrillation, *Acta Cardiol* 1981; **36**: 431–44.

32. Graboys TB, Podrid PJ, Lown B, Efficacy of amiodarone for refractory supraventricular tachyarrhythmias, *Am Heart J* 1983; **106**: 870–6.

33. Gosselink AM, Crijns HJ, Isabelle CVG, Hillige H, Wiesfeld ACP, Lie KI, Low dose amiodarone for maintenance of sinus rhythm after cardioversion of atrial fibrillation or atrial flutter, *JAMA* 1992; **267**: 3289–93.

34. Acquati F, Forgione F, Caico S et al, Prophylaxis of atrial fibrillation following electrical cardioversion. A prospective randomised study comparing low-dose and very low-dose amiodarone to propafenone: preliminary results, *J Am Coll Cardiol* 1997; **29**: 112A.

35. Gold RL, Haffajee CL, Charos G, Solan K, Baker S, Alpert JS, Amiodarone for refractory atrial fibrillation, *Am J Cardiol* 1986; **57**: 124–7.

36. Horowitz LN, Spielman SR, Greenspan AM et al, Use of amiodarone in persistent and paroxysmal atrial fibrilation resistant to quinidine therapy, *J Am Coll Cardiol* 1985; **6**: 1402–7.

37. Amiodarone Trials Meta-analysis Investigators. Effect of prophylactic amiodarone on mortality after acute myocardial infarction and in congestive heart failure: meta-analysis of individual data from 6500 patients in randomised trials, *Lancet* 1997; **350**: 1417–24.

38. The DIAMOND Study Group, Dofetilide in patients with left ventricular dysfunction and either heart failure or acute myocardial infarction: rationale, design, and patient characteristics of the DIAMOND studies, *Clin Cardiol* 1997; **20**: 704–10.

39. Danish Trial in Acute Myocardial Infarction on Dofetilide (DIAMOND), Preliminary results presented at the European Congress of Cardiology, Stockholm, 1997.

40. Prystowsky EN, Benson DW, Fuster V et al, Management of patients with atrial fibrillation. A statement for healthcare professionals from the committee on electrocardiography and electrophysiology, American Heart Association, *Circulation* 1996; **93**: 1262–77.

41. Gardner MJ, Gilbert M, Heart rate control in patients with atrial fibrillation, *Can J Cardiol* 1996; **12**: 21A–23A.

42. Cosio FG, Lopez-Gil M, Goicolea A et al, Radiofrequency ablation of the inferior vena cava-tricuspid valve isthmus in common atrial flutter, *Am J Cardiol* 1993; **71**: 705–9.

43. Cairns JA, Atrial fibrillation: antithrombotic therapy. In: Yusuf S, Cairns JA, Camm AJ, Fallen EL, Gersh BJ, eds, *Evidence based Cardiology.* (BMJ Books: London, 1998) 544–52.

44. Atrial fibrillation Investigators, Risk factors for stroke and efficiency of antithrombotic therapy in atrial fibrillation. Analysis of pooled data from five randomised controlled trials, *Arch Intern Med* 1994; **154**: 1449–57.

45. Krikler DM, Perelman M, Rowland E, Mandel WJ, Ventricular tachycardia and ventricular fibrillation. In: Mandel WJ, ed., *Cardiac Arrhythmias. Their Mechanisms, Diagnosis, and Management* (J. B. Lippincott: Philadelphia, 1995) 649–91.

46. Adgey AAJ, Allen JD, Geddes JS et al, Acute myocardial infarction, *Lancet* 1971; **ii**: 501–4.

47. Antman EM, Berlin JA, Declining incidence of ventricular fibrillation in myocardial infarction, *Circulation* 1992; **86**: 764–73.

48. Campbell RWF, Murray A, Julian D, Ventricular arrhythmias in the first 12 hours of acute myocardial infarction. Natural history study, *Br Heart J* 1981; **46**: 351–7.

49. Wolfe CL, Nibley C, Bhandari A et al, Polymorphic ventricular tachycardia associated with acute myocardial infarction, *Circulation* 1991; **84**: 1543–51.

50. Echt DS, Liebson PR, Mitchell LB et al, Mortality and morbidity in patients receiving encanide, fleccanide or placebo. The Cardiac Arrhythmia Suppression Trial, *N Engl J Med* 1991; **324**: 781–7.

51. Waldo AL, Camm AJ, deRuyter H et al, Effect of d-sotalol on mortality in patients with left ventricular dysfunction after recent and remote myocardial infarction, *Lancet* 1996; **348**: 7–12.

52. Touboul P, Moleur P, Mathieu MP et al, A comparative evaluation of the effects of propafenone and lidocaine on early ventricular arrhythmias after acute myocardial infarction, *Eur Heart J* 1988; **9**: 1188–93

53. Silke B, Frais MA, Verma SP et al, Comparative haemodynamic effects of propafenone and lidocaine on early ventricular arrhythmias after acute myocardial infarction, *Br J Clin Pharmacol* 1986; **22**: 707–14.

54. Ronnevik PK, Gundersen T, Abrahamsen AM, Tolerability and antiarrhythmic efficacy of disopyramide compared to lignocaine in selected patients with suspected acute myocardial infarction, *Eur Heart J* 1987; **8**: 19–24.

55. The AVID Investigators, A comparison of antiarrhythmic drug therapy with implantable defibrillators in patients resuscitated from near fatal ventricular arrhythmias, *N Engl J Med* 1997; **337**: 1576–83.

56. Siebels J, Cappato R, Ruppel R et al,

Preliminary results of the Cardiac Arrest Study Hamburg (CASH), *Am J Cardiol* 1993; 72(suppl): 109F–13F.

57. Connolly SJ, Gent M, Roberts RS et al, Canadian Implantable Defibrillators Study (CIDS): study design and organisation, *Am J Cardiol* 1993; 72(suppl): 103F–8F.

58. La Rovere MT, Bigger JT Jr, Marcus FI, Mortara A, Schwartz PJ, for the ATRAMI (Autonomic Tone and Reflexes After Myocardial Infarction) Investigators, Baroreflex sensitivity and heart-rate variability in prediction of total cardiac mortality after myocardial infarction, *Lancet* 1998; 35: 478–84.

59. Beta-blocker Heart Attack Trial Research Group, A randomised trial of propranolol in patients with acute myocardial infarction, *JAMA* 1982; 247: 1701–14.

60. The Norwegian Multicentre Study Group, Timolol-induced reduction in mortality and reinfarction in patients surviving acute myocardial infarction, *Lancet* 1979; 11: 865–72.

61. Hjalmarson A, Elmfeldt D, Herlitz J et al, Effect on mortality of metoprolol in acute myocardial infarction. A double-blind randomised trial, *Lancet* 1981; 1: 823–7.

62. The Cardiac Arrhythmia Suppression Trial II Investigators, Effect of the anti-arrhythmic agent moricizine on survival after myocardial infarction, *N Engl J Med* 1992; 327: 227–33.

63. Cairns JA, Connolly SJ, Roberts R, Gent M, for the Canadian Amiodarone Myocardial

Infarction Arrhythmia Trial investigators, Randomised trial of outcome after myocardial infarction in patients with frequent or repetitive ventricular premature depolarisations: CAMIAT, *Lancet* 1997; 349: 675–82.

64. Julian D, Camm AJ, Frangin G, et al, Randomised trial of effect of amiodarone on mortality in patients with left-ventricular dysfunction after recent myocardial infarction: EMIAT, *Lancet* 1997; 349: 667–74.

65. Moss AJ, Hall WJ, Cannom DS et al, Improved survival with an implantable defibrillator in patients with coronary artery disease at high risk for ventricular arrhythmias, *N Engl J Med* 1996; 335: 1933–40.

66. Bigger JT, for the CABG-Patch Trial Investigators, Prophylactic use of implanted cardiac defibrillators in patients at high risk for ventricular arrhythmias after coronary artery bypass graft surgery, *N Engl J Med* 1997; 337: 1569–75.

67. Connolly SJ, Non-pharmacologic therapy for sustained ventricular tachycardia and ventricular fibrillation. In: Yusuf S, Cairns JA, Camm AJ, Fallen EL, Gersh BJ, eds, *Evidence based Cardiology*. (BMJ Books: London, 1998) 586–95.

68. Buxton AE, Fisher JD, Josephson ME at al, Prevention of sudden death in patients with coronary artery disease. The Multicenter Unsustained Tachycardia Trial (MUSST), *Prog Cardiovasc Dis* 1993; 36: 215–26.

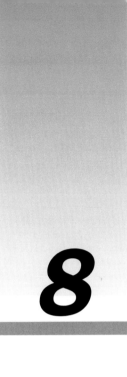

Surgery for coronary artery disease

Samer A M Nashef

The heart is a pump. When it goes wrong, the cause is usually valve malfunction, pipe blockage or pump failure. All of these are mechanical problems which should have mechanical or surgical solutions. From this viewpoint, it is surprising that surgery for heart disease remained virtually non-existent before the second half of this century, and coronary surgery did not start in earnest until the second half of the 1960s. The obstacles responsible for this delay in the development of heart surgery give valuable insights into the state of the art today and the problems in store for tomorrow.

History

A late developer

While surgeons were making great strides in other fields, cardiac surgery stayed in abeyance because of two apparently insurmountable problems. To carry out a heart operation under ideal conditions, the heart must be motionless (for a technically satisfactory result) and bloodless (to prevent exsanguination). But a motionless heart for any length of time results in a dead patient, and a heart deprived of blood supply dies itself, with the same end result. Two questions therefore had to be addressed before cardiac surgery could begin to evolve: how to keep the patient alive while the heart is being operated on, and how to keep the heart itself alive while it is being operated on. Some heart operations were possible in a beating, full heart. Closed mitral valvotomy, for example, could be carried out 'blind', by inserting a finger or an instrument into the left atrium or ventricle to stretch, cut or tear open the fused rheumatic, stenotic valve. Coronary arteries, however, are smaller, more delicate and far less forgiving, and coronary surgery had to wait until the prerequisite of a bloodless, motionless heart could be reliably and safely achieved.

Protect and survive

The pioneers explored two approaches simultaneously. Hypothermia, achieved by plunging the anaesthetized patient into an ice bath, could lengthen the time for which the circulation could be safely stopped. Extracorporeal circulation, by temporarily perfusing the body from an external heart–lung machine, could maintain tissue perfusion and oxygenation despite an arrested heart. Both had limited success in the early years, and cardiac surgery developed by using both together for added safety. Once it was shown that heart surgery could be carried out relatively safely using these techniques, the way was clear for the development of coronary surgery.

Sideways moves

The relationship between the symptom of angina and stenotic coronary arteries was well established. Early attempts at a surgical solution could not directly tackle the coronary arteries themselves because of the problems discussed above. However, to many innovators, the lack of a safe way to operate directly on the heart was no bar to the development of a number of operations for angina. Some of these operations were ingenious and many were absurd, but all testified to the inventiveness and powers of lateral thinking of their originators. Examples of such operations were aortic or coronary sympathectomy (to cut the nerve pathways of angina), internal mammary artery ligation (to 'encourage' more blood to go to the pericardium rather than the chest wall) and pericardial abrasion with muscle flap transfer[1] (to stimulate the development of collateral vessels). Perhaps the most well known of these is the Vineberg procedure,[2] in which the internal mammary artery was taken down from the chest wall and divided distally. Its bleeding cut end was then implanted into the wall of the left ventricle, close to the left anterior descending (LAD) coronary artery, in the hope that collaterals would develop between the two vessels.

Cardiopulmonary bypass

The overwhelming majority of cardiac and coronary operations rely on the heart–lung machine. This piece of equipment (Fig. 8.1) looks daunting and complex at first, but its essential components are simple. It consists of a pump (the heart substitute) and an oxygenator (the lung substitute). The pump is usually a roller-type device in which a circulating roller squeezes sections of flexible plastic tubing to propel the blood forward. The oxygenator provides a surface (usually a membrane) across which gas exchange can take place. To prepare the patient for extracorporeal circulation, a cannula is

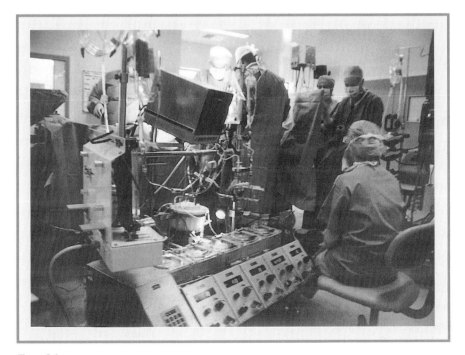

Figure 8.1
The heart–lung machine in action. The perfusionist is seated in the foreground, monitoring a bank of five roller pumps, each with separate flow controls. One supplies arterial return to the patient. Two others provide suction to return any spilt blood to the heart–lung machine and thence back to the patient to minimize blood loss. The large container in front of the roller pumps is the oxygenator to which venous blood is drained from the patient. The two tubes rising towards the patient are the arterial and venous lines.

inserted into the right atrium and another into the aorta. The right atrial cannula collects venous return into the oxygenator where gas exchange takes place. The blood, thus oxygenated, is then returned to the patient by the pump through the aortic cannula. When the circuit is established and running, the ventilator can be switched off and the heart can be stopped with relative safety. The heart and lungs are now effectively bypassed, and this is often referred to by patients as a 'heart bypass operation'. The second use of the term 'bypass' is an abbreviation of coronary artery *bypass* grafting. This dual meaning in such a small field is unfortunate.

Myocardial protection

During cardiopulmonary bypass, the heart beats largely empty. The coronary arteries are, however, still being perfused from the aorta, which itself receives its supply from the heart–lung machine. Opening the coronary arteries in this setting results in a gush of blood which makes surgery on them difficult. If, however, the aorta is clamped between the site of insertion of the aortic cannula and the origin of the coronary arteries, a bloodless field becomes possible. The disadvantage, of course, is that the heart is now globally ischaemic. In this context, it is best to think of ischaemia as an imbalance between oxygen supply and demand. During aortic clamping, oxygen supply is nil. The heart can then be

protected by reducing oxygen demand to as close to nil as possible. This is achieved in several ways. Oxygen requirements are already reduced by the fact that the empty heart, though beating, is not actually working (preload and afterload reduction). If hypothermic bypass is being used, oxygen requirements are lower still. Finally, the infusion of a cold, high-potassium solution into the coronary arteries further lowers the temperature of the myocardium and produces cardiac standstill. Under these conditions, the empty, cold and motionless heart will survive with virtually no clinically detectable damage for about an hour. This is ample time for most heart operations. The solution in question is appropriately termed 'cardioplegia' or 'cardioplegic solution'. There are many recipes for its composition, its temperature and the method, frequency and site of its administration, but the key ingredient is potassium.

(An alternative approach to cardioplegia is to carry out the operation using several short, unprotected periods of ischaemia. This is done by clamping the aorta, and fibrillating the heart for a few minutes during which a segment of saphenous vein is sutured to a coronary artery (the distal anastomosis). The aorta is unclamped, allowing the heart to recover from ischaemia while the vein is sutured to the aorta (the proximal anastomosis). The process is then repeated for subsequent bypass grafts. This method, called 'cross-clamp fibrillation', is popular in some London hospitals.)

Coronary artery bypass grafting (CABG)

Favoloro first described the use of saphenous vein to bypass a diseased coronary artery in 1968.[3] Since that time, CABG has become the commonest operation for ischaemic heart disease and one of the most commonly performed surgical operations worldwide. It is also the most studied, documented, evaluated and audited therapy in the history of medicine.

Indications

There are two broad indications for CABG: symptomatic and prognostic. The symptomatic indication is straightforward: it is angina which is not satisfactorily controlled by medical treatment. The prognostic indication is the presence of disease which has been shown to have a better prognosis with surgery than with medical therapy. Such disease, in descending order of prognostic importance, includes the following:

- significant (>50%) stenosis of the main stem of the left coronary artery;
- significant (>50%) proximal stenosis of the three major coronary arteries: the

LAD, circumflex and right coronary arteries;
- significant (>50%) stenosis of two major coronary arteries, including high-grade stenosis of the proximal LAD.

The presence of impaired left ventricular function increases the prognostic advantage of surgery over medical treatment in all categories.

The decision to go ahead with CABG should normally be taken by the patient, armed with the necessary information to make that decision. This information allows the patient to weigh the benefits of the operation against the risks. The primary benefit of the operation is the disappearance of the symptom of angina. This is a reliable outcome, as more than 95% of patients who undergo CABG can expect their angina to disappear completely after surgery. In addition, there are prognostic advantages depending on the nature and distribution of the disease. For example, a patient with severe angina and triple-vessel disease can expect to benefit both symptomatically and prognostically from operation, whereas a patient with no angina but with left main stem stenosis and poor left ventricular function should seriously consider having the operation on prognostic grounds alone. The patient with no angina and only single vessel disease not affecting the proximal LAD should not be offered surgery. Much of this information is obtained from an extensive list of publications derived from two major randomized studies of coronary surgery: the American CASS (Coronary Artery Surgery Study) and the European Coronary Surgery Study. Early reports from these studies showed the symptomatic advantages of coronary surgery over medical treatment.[4,5] As follow-up lengthened with time, the prognostic advantages began to emerge in a number of categories.

Once the benefits of surgery are established, they need to be weighed against the risks. The mortality for CABG in the absence of any risk factors is only 0.36%.[6] Many risk factors, however, increase this figure, so that overall mortality for all coronary surgery in the UK is between 2% and 4%. Risk factors that contribute to higher mortality after CABG are age, female sex, impaired left ventricular function, severe pulmonary, neurological and renal dysfunction, extracardiac arteriopathy and emergency or repeat operation. There are elaborate risk stratification methods[7,8] for the assessment of approximate risk in individual patients and these can be consulted to provide a 'quote' or an estimate of mortality, adjusted for the actual results of the individual surgeon and institution in question. Decisions are made somewhat more difficult because of the coronary surgery paradox: the higher the risk of operation, the greater is the advantage of surgical over medical treatment.[9]

Investigations

Coronary angiography remains the essential investigation for patients before CABG. It is important because it determines the site of the stenoses and therefore the number and target positions of the bypass grafts needed. At the same time, left ventricular angiography gives an indication of left ventricular function.

The operation

For the purposes of this narrative we shall assume a typical, low-risk patient: he is male, in his late sixties, with angina and triple-vessel coronary artery disease. He is anaesthetized and intubated for ventilation. A radial artery cannula is inserted for continuous monitoring of blood pressure and blood gas sampling. A catheter is inserted through the internal jugular vein into the right atrium to monitor central venous pressure and to allow access for the administration of vasoactive drugs. The bladder is also catheterized.

After skin preparation and draping, a member of the surgical team incises the leg to harvest the saphenous vein, while another surgeon simultaneously opens the chest by median sternotomy. The left half of the sternum is then elevated to allow access to the left internal mammary artery (LIMA), which is taken down from the chest wall with a combination of sharp dissection and

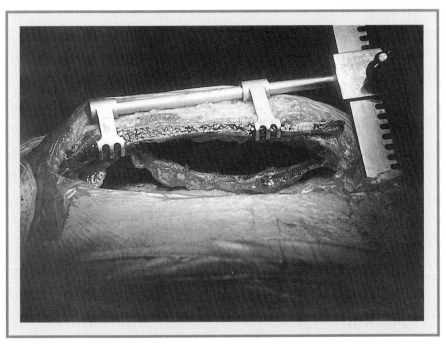

Figure 8.2
Sternotomy and internal mammary artery harvest. Surgeon's view from the right-hand side of the patient. The sternum is divided and its left half is elevated by the claws of a retractor. Most of the left internal mammary artery (LIMA) has been dissected from the chest wall, but the proximal quarter is still to be done. The LIMA has been taken down as a pedicle, incorporating its accompanying veins and surrounding soft tissue. This is to avoid surgical injury to the fragile arterial wall. The left pleural space is wide open and can be seen behind the LIMA pedicle.

electrocautery (Fig. 8.2). The branches of the LIMA are clipped or coagulated. The tributaries of the long saphenous vein are ligated.

Once the conduits are ready, the patient is fully anticoagulated with heparin and the heart is prepared for cardiopulmonary bypass. To achieve this, purse-string sutures are placed in the ascending aorta and right atrium. These are used to secure the aortic or arterial cannula, which brings oxygenated blood from the heart–lung machine to the aorta, and the right atrial or venous cannula which drains

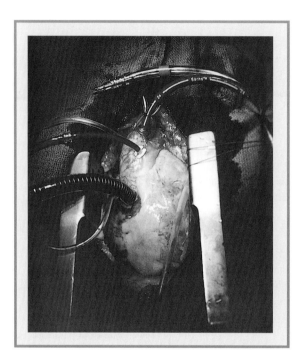

Figure 8.3
Cannulation for cardiopulmonary bypass. Direct overview of the sternotomy. The topmost, free tube with a band is a vent tube to be used later to keep the heart empty of blood. Below that, the aortic or arterial cannula is into the aorta, and below it the cannula for delivering cardioplegic solution (the aortic clamp will be applied between these two cannulae). The large, wire-reinforced cannula to the left of the picture is the venous cannula which is positioned in the right atrium. Both the venous and arterial cannulae are secured by purse-string sutures held in tubular snuggers. The arterial cannula has two of these for extra security. The finer tube to the right is a pericardial sucker, returning any spilt blood to the heart–lung machine. Most of what is visible of the heart here is the right ventricle with its covering of epicardial fat.

deoxygenated blood from the right atrium to the heart–lung machine (Fig. 8.3).

Cardiopulmonary bypass is begun by unclamping the right atrial cannula, allowing deoxygenated blood freely to siphon down into the oxygenator where gas exchange takes place. The blood is then pumped into the aorta through the arterial cannula. For the first few seconds, only pump priming fluid is infused into the patient, but within 1 min the heart–lung machine is normally pumping oxygenated blood at the usual cardiac output of 5 litres or so per minute (cardiac index of 2.4). Once that is established, the patient will survive without cardiac or pulmonary function, and the ventilator is now switched off.

The surgeon then assesses the targets for grafting. In the right coronary territory, the target is usually the distal right coronary artery (RCA) or its main branch, the posterior descending (PD) artery. The circumflex coronary artery is hidden posteriorly in the atrioventricular groove and relatively inaccessible; its major branch, the first obtuse marginal (OM), is usually chosen for grafting. The LAD is also chosen, and one of its diagonal branches may also be separately grafted. The surgeon normally selects the first healthy segment of the coronary artery (assessed by look and feel) beyond the stenosis (located by angiography) as the target for the conduit.

Once the targets have been identified, the aorta is clamped and cardioplegic solution is infused rapidly into the aortic root. The solution cannot flow distally into the aortic arch because of the clamp and it cannot flow proximally into the left ventricle because of the aortic valve: the only flow is therefore into the coronary arteries. The heart normally stops within 30 s to 1 min of the beginning of cardioplegic infusion, and the operation can begin.

The surgeon then makes a longitudinal arteriotomy (about 5 mm long) in the distal RCA or PD to which the cut end of a length of saphenous vein is sutured with a fine monofilament suture, usually 7/0 polypropylene (Fig. 8.4). Another length of saphenous vein is then similarly sutured to the OM arteriotomy. The cut end of the LIMA is then sutured to the LAD arteriotomy (Fig. 8.5). The part of the operation that needs a still, bloodless heart is now over, and the aortic clamp is removed, allowing blood to flow down the coronary arteries. This washes out the cardioplegic solution and perfuses the heart, which then starts to beat. Each coronary anastomosis takes 5–15 min to fashion. The overall time during which the heart is ischaemic in a triple CABG therefore varies between 15 and 45 min, well within the ischaemic tolerance of a heart relaxed by cardioplegia. This period is called the 'cross-clamp time' and is measured and recorded in all heart operations.

The LIMA graft is now functional. The vein grafts, however, need an arterial blood source at their proximal ends. To achieve this, a segment of aorta is isolated in a partially occluding clamp and small incisions or circular punch holes are made in that segment. The ends of the vein grafts are then sutured to these with a fine monofilament suture (typically 6/0 polypropylene). The clamp is removed and the vein grafts are now functional.

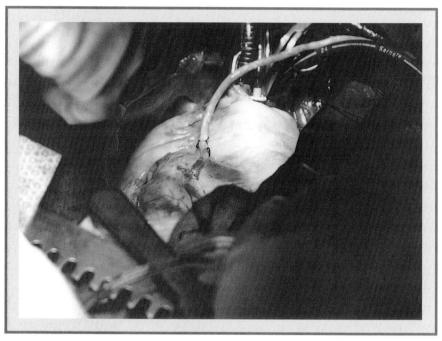

Figure 8.4
Right coronary artery graft. Left caudal view, with the heart rotated to expose the right margin. A segment of saphenous vein has been sutured to an arteriotomy in the right coronary artery. The vein will be later cut to size and its other end sutured to the ascending aorta.

The time has now come to disconnect the patient from the heart–lung machine. The ventilator is restarted. The perfusionist then slowly and gradually occludes the right atrial cannula, allowing more blood to enter the heart, while simultaneously reducing the flow of the pump. The heart gradually takes over the circulation and the right atrial cannula is fully clamped and removed. The total time of extracorporeal circulation is typically between 30 and 75 min, and this time is also measured and recorded as the 'bypass time'.

The effects of heparin are then reversed with protamine and the arterial cannula is removed. Haemostasis is secured, chest drains are inserted and the chest is closed with stainless steel wires for the sternum and

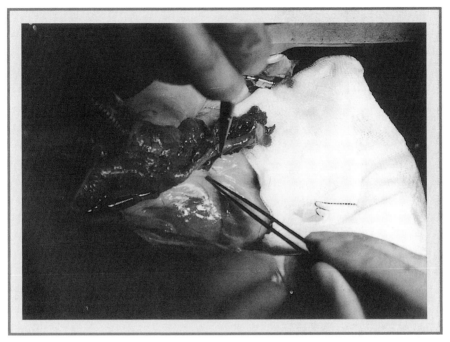

Figure 8.5
Left anterior descending (LAD) coronary artery graft. Surgeon's eye view, from the right-hand side of the patient. A thick pedicle containing the left internal mammary artery (LIMA) lies on the surface of the heart. The LIMA is being sutured to the LAD. The small, metallic 'bulldog' clamp occludes the LIMA until the anastomosis is complete. Once the LIMA-to-LAD anastomosis is done, the aortic clamp is released, allowing bloodflow down the native coronary arteries. The heart then resumes beating. In the background, a saphenous vein graft to the obtuse marginal branch of the circumflex coronary artery has already been completed.

sutures for the soft tissues and the skin. The patient is then transferred to a critical care area for postoperative monitoring.

Postoperative course

The patient is monitored for overall cardiac and haemodynamic function, respiratory function and bleeding. Once all parameters are stable (1–6 h after return from theatre), anaesthesia is stopped and the patient wakes up and is extubated. Overnight monitoring continues until the morning of the first postoperative day (day 1), when the chest drains and radial cannula are removed and the patient returned to the ward. Oral intake is encouraged and, if adequate, the central venous line and urinary catheter are removed on day 2. The patient walks on day 3, climbs stairs on day 4 or 5 and is normally ready for discharge from day 6. Heavy use of the upper arm and shoulder muscles is discouraged until the sternum has fully healed (2–3 months). All other physical activity is permissible provided the patient feels up to it. Most patients are back to normal and fully active within the first 6 weeks.

Complications

CABG is a now a common operation. It is, nevertheless, a major invasive procedure with many attendant risks. The relatively low rate of major complications pays tribute to the efforts of the many surgeons, anaesthetists, perfusionists and nurses who have worked tirelessly towards reducing the risk of this intervention. 'Low complications', however, will never become 'no complications'. The following is a list, with brief descriptions, of the adverse events of CABG.

Bleeding

At the end of a CABG operation, there are several vascular anastomoses, aortic and atrial cannulation sites, some 20 or so LIMA branches, another 20 or so saphenous vein tributaries, an incised pericardium and a divided and bloody sternum. All this is against a background of severe platelet dysfunction because of cardiopulmonary bypass, preoperative aspirin administration or both. Although a degree of coagulaopathy is probably desirable in fine vascular anastomoses because of the risk of graft thrombosis, it undoubtedly contributes to postoperative bleeding. Most patients will lose at least 200–600 ml of blood through the drains in the first 12 h, and this is to be expected. When bleeding is excessive, however, the chest must be re-explored to exclude or treat a surgical cause. Between 1% and 4% of patients return to theatre for re-exploration for bleeding after CABG, almost all within 12 h of operation.

Atrial dysrhythmias

Atrial fibrillation or flutter occur in 10–40% of patients after CABG. The reason for this is not fully understood, but a combination of factors may contribute to this incidence. These include the abrupt withdrawal of beta-blockers and other anti-anginal medication, the surgical manipulation of the right atrium and possibly inadequate protection of the conduction system during myocardial ischaemic time. Such arrhythmias can occur at any time up to 4 weeks after CABG but the peak incidence is on days 3 and 4. This complication is benign, but is often poorly tolerated by the patient, increases postoperative tiredness and undoubtedly delays hospital discharge. It is also a main cause of readmission to hospital after CABG. Treatment policies vary. Most surgeons agree that serum potassium should be kept above 4.5, and correction of a lower serum potassium concentration may suffice to convert the patient back to sinus rhythm. If the arrhythmia persists, it may be treated with digoxin, low-dose beta-blockade, amiodarone or cardioversion. Warfarin must be considered for atrial fibrillation that persists beyond 48–72 h.

Infection and wound problems

Leg wound problems are very common after CABG. Small areas of superficial infection, scab formation and delayed healing probably occur in a third of patients, giving rise to the well-known aphorism 'Coronary surgery is a pain in the leg!' Sternal wound problems are thankfully less frequent but much more serious. Occasional superficial infection and delayed healing may occur, but the development of deep infection may lead to mediastinitis and sternal wound dehiscence. This occurs in approximately 2% of patients, with diabetes, obesity and internal mammary artery harvest the predominant risk factors. With the increase in the prevalence of methicillin-resistant organisms, treatment of this condition is becoming more difficult. It

usually involves return to theatre with surgical debridement, rewiring and mediastinal irrigation. Sometimes plastic surgical procedures are also needed. As expected, mediastinitis with sternal dehiscence carries a significant mortality, particularly in the elderly.

After CABG, there is often an area of numbness anterior to the leg wound resulting from the manipulation of the saphenous nerve, which is closely applied to the saphenous vein. There is also an area of paraesthesia over the mammary artery bed, which sometimes becomes hypersensitive and dysaesthetic. This usually resolves with time, but may persist for a few months in some patients. In a tiny minority of patients, paraesthesia turns into a chronic debilitating pain which needs the services of a pain clinic.

Cerebral complications

Stroke is a rare but distinct possibility. It may be caused by embolism of atheromatous debris from the ascending aorta, of air from opening sections of the aorta and coronary arteries and of platelets and other microemboli from the heart–lung machine. Patients with coronary artery disease may have atheromatous disease elsewhere, and severe cerebrovascular disease will predispose to hypoperfusion strokes during the operation. The risk factors for this complication are age and extracardiac arteriopathy. Although frank, irreversible stroke is rare, most patients have some degree of neurological impairment after CABG on psychometric testing. The tests return to normal after a few weeks.

Long-term outcome

Most patients return to a normal, angina-free lifestyle, with a reduced risk of adverse cardiac events and a correspondingly increased survival. This happy state of affairs continues for many years but is not permanent. Although CABG is a 'definitive' operation in most elderly patients, some, particularly younger, patients may experience a return of angina. When this happens, it is typically 10–12 years after the original operation but may occur only a few weeks postoperatively in some unfortunate individuals. Recurrent angina may be due to progression of the native disease, so that new stenoses appear in ungrafted, previously healthy coronary arteries or in previously grafted coronary arteries beyond the site of implantation of the graft. The LIMA, if patent the morning after the operation, is likely to remain so indefinitely. Unfortunately, this is not true of saphenous vein grafts: they have an attrition rate due to a combination of thrombotic occlusion (early) or to the development of vein graft disease (late). Veins were never 'designed' to be arteries, and most will, sooner or later, develop intimal hyperplasia with smooth

muscle proliferation leading to stenosis and finally occlusion. A reasonable estimate is that around 50% of vein grafts will have occluded by 12 years. Patients with one or two occluded vein grafts may nevertheless continue to do well because of other patent grafts, in particular the LIMA. Those who develop symptoms should be assessed and investigated as usual. They may be offered, as appropriate, medical treatment, angioplasty or repeat CABG. If the last option is being contemplated, the additional risk of a repeat operation should be taken into account when the decision is made.

New developments

The success and long-term patency of the LIMA as a conduit for CABG has stimulated a search for other arterial conduits in the hope of achieving superior patency rates over saphenous vein grafts. The right internal mammary artery, the gastroepiploic artery and the inferior epigastric artery have all been used with varying degrees of success. Recently, there has been a revival of the use of the radial artery as a conduit, and many surgeons now use it in preference to saphenous vein. Early patency rates appear encouraging and we await the results of randomized control trials of radial artery versus saphenous vein with great interest.

Transmyocardial revascularization (TMR) is a technique in which laser beams are used to drill channels through the myocardium into the left ventricular cavity. If these channels stay patent, they may provide a communication between the left ventricle and the intramyocardial sinusoids, allowing direct perfusion of the myocardium from the left ventricle itself. Such perfusion is known to exist in some reptilian hearts. There are anecdotal reports of success of this technique but it has not yet been fully evaluated. The results of a randomized controlled trial recently carried out in Cambridge have not been encouraging.[10] The operation is normally carried out through a left thoracotomy, but recently available equipment permits a percutaneous, endoluminal approach, transferring this procedure to the domain of the interventional cardiologists.

Minimally invasive surgery has been attempted in various forms. At one end of the spectrum, percutaneous cardiopulmonary bypass with endoscopic conduit harvesting allows for a full, multigraft operation to be carried out without dividing the sternum. This relies on a large array of expensive, disposable equipment and is time-consuming, but has the potential of truly replacing the conventional CABG operation. There is even an attempt at replacing the surgeon's hands within the chest with small, robotic hands controlled by the surgeon from outside, another room or even another continent! At the other end of the spectrum, a simple operation to anastomose the LIMA to the

LAD on the beating heart can be carried out through a small incision in the anterior left chest. This can be performed with little more than the standard instruments for minor surgery, with or without contraptions to help steady the heart. Provided the patient has only single-vessel disease and the topography is favourable, this operation, without cardiopulmonary bypass, is almost a minor procedure which may compete with angioplasty in the future. The number of patients suitable for this approach is, however, limited. Combinations of the above techniques with angioplasty are also being evaluated.

Surgery for the broken heart

CABG is the main operation for coronary artery disease and is directed at the coronary arteries themselves. There are, however, complications of myocardial infarction which result in mechanical cardiac problems which are best dealt with surgically. When infarction occurs, part of the heart muscle dies and is replaced by fibrous scar tissue. If that segment of myocardium breaks down before healing and scarring takes place, a number of conditions may occur, depending on the site of the infarct.

Cardiac rupture

If the infarct is in the free wall of the left ventricle, cardiac rupture occurs. This condition, often rapidly fatal, is fortunately rare. If the patient survives, the presenting feature is that of cardiac tamponade. The rupture may well have sealed by the time of presentation, so that pericardial drainage is all that is required. If the rupture has not sealed, a limited operation for surgical closure may be indicated. The recently infarcted heart tolerates surgery badly, and the tissues are often too friable for suturing. The outcome is poor, with a mortality rate between 20% and 50%.

Ventricular septal rupture

If the infarct is in the septum, acute postinfarction septal rupture may result. The two arteries that supply the septum are the LAD (through its septal branches) and the RCA (through the septal branches of its posterior descending branch). It therefore follows that the septal rupture may be anterior (in LAD occlusion) or inferior (in RCA occlusion). Typically, the patient who is recovering satisfactorily from myocardial infarction develops sudden deterioration 5–10 days after the infarct. Examination reveals a prominent right ventricular impulse with a harsh systolic murmur. Depending on the size of the left-to-right shunt, there may be pulmonary oedema, shock or acute renal failure. The diagnosis can be confirmed by echocardiography or right heart catheterization (to demonstrate a rise in

oxygen saturation between the right atrium and pulmonary artery, indicating a shunt at the level of the ventricle). Both investigations will distinguish septal rupture from mitral rupture, which has a similar presentation (see below). The surgical management of ventricular septal rupture is controversial. There are no randomized trials to guide us and most surgeons have evolved policies based on a combination of common sense, experience and prejudice. The following two paragraphs will relate, respectively, what is common sense and what is prejudice (the author's, necessarily!).

Those patients in a critical state, with shock, acute renal failure and pulmonary oedema will die without surgery, yet they have the highest risk from surgery. Intra-aortic balloon counterpulsation will improve the condition of these patients, but only temporarily and incompletely: they remain critically ill, even on the balloon. Early operation has poorer results, partly because of the friability of tissues and the recency of the infarct. Delayed operation has better results, partly because of the above, but also because of self-selection: the most critical will have died waiting. The fragile heart, already suffering from a recent ischaemic insult, will be grateful for a quick operation with minimal ischaemia. Concomitant CABG may not be in the patient's best interests. If, however, there is coronary disease with a prognostic implication, the patient may survive the operation only to die from anther infarct soon afterwards. Whether coronary angiography is needed depends on the surgical policy. A surgeon who has no intention of performing concomitant CABG is probably happier not seeing the state of the coronary arteries. The outcome is related to right ventricular function: this unfortunate chamber, already suffering from an ischaemic insult (the myocardial infarct), is now subject to a pressure injury (the force of LV pressure) and to overwork abuse (substantially higher flow because of the shunt). The worse the function of the right ventricle, the poorer is the outcome. Inferior septal rupture has a worse prognosis. Finally, if the patient is (miraculously) asymptomatic with a postinfarct septal rupture and the defect is well tolerated by all organ systems, delaying the operation by 6 weeks will allow for elective and safe surgery with a predictably good result. On this most surgeons agree.

My view is that coronary angiography is worthwhile, so that major coronary arteries with high-grade stenoses can be grafted. Emergency operation is crucial for survival in all patients with the exception of those not at all compromised by the rupture (see above). The intra-aortic balloon counterpulsation pump is useful in supporting some patients from diagnosis to operation, but must not be used as a holding measure to delay operation.

Most of the operation can be carried out without clamping the aorta, and judicious use of any vein grafts, by connecting them to the heart–lung machine, allows perfusion of the ischaemic myocardium immediately and during any periods of aortic clamping. The friability of the heart is tackled by 'wallpapering' the entire septum with a pericardial patch, loosely sutured from the LV side, so that the LV pressure pastes the patch onto the septum. This deals with most of the concerns regarding immediate operation. Of course, on this, many surgeons disagree.

Mitral rupture

If the infarct destroys a papillary muscle supporting the mitral valve, rupture can result with severe mitral regurgitation. Typically, the patient who is recovering satisfactorily from myocardial infarction develops sudden deterioration 5–10 days after the infarct. Examination reveals a harsh pan-systolic murmur in the mitral area. There may be pulmonary oedema, shock and acute renal failure. If this sounds familiar, it should (see ventricular septal rupture, above). This condition is even worse than septal rupture, with few survivors beyond 24 h and almost none beyond 30 days without operation. Echocardiography or right heart catheterization establish the diagnosis and help distinguish between mitral and septal rupture. Treatment is by urgent or emergency mitral valve repair or replacement, and the controversies regarding timing of operation and the desirability of concomitant CABG also apply here.

Left ventricular aneurysm

Sometimes, an anterior or, less frequently, an inferior infarct turns into a thinned-out fibrous scar, an aneurysm, which enlarges with time. This creates a 'dead space' which moves paradoxically with cardiac contraction and, depending on its size, may severely compromise the efficiency of ejection. The patient may present with tiredness, shortness of breath or heart failure. The aneurysm can be surgically resected, usually but not always in conjunction with CABG, leaving a smaller but fitter heart. Left ventricular aneurysmectomy is carried out in 1–5% of CABG operations. The risk increase is marginal and the benefits are those of improving dyspnoea and reducing the risk of heart failure, further aneurysmal expansion and thromboembolism.

The last resort

The improvement in surgical techniques and results has meant that ischaemic hearts can be treated surgically even in the presence of severe impairment of myocardial function. There comes a time, however, when the ravages of ischaemia are such that there is no

further reversible change and the heart is so weakened by infarction that the predominant symptom is no longer the anginal pain of ischaemic muscle but the dyspnoea and congestive failure of long-dead muscle. At that point, the only surgical option is heart replacement. Today, cardiac transplantation offers a realistic therapy for selected patients with end-stage coronary artery disease where the main problem is failure of the pump itself. Patients with ischaemic heart disease represent about 55% of those on the waiting list for heart transplantation. The restricted availability of donor hearts clearly limits the widespread use of this therapy, but the results are good, with 1-year and 5-year survival approaching 90% and 70% respectively, with an excellent quality of life. The long-term complications are related to infection, because of the use of immunosuppressant drugs, and rejection, which is often manifested by accelerated coronary disease in the transplanted heart. The limited supply of donor organs has stimulated work into other forms of cardiac replacement such as xenotransplantation and permanent, artificial hearts.

References

1.   Beck CS, The development of a new blood supply to the heart by operation, *Ann Surg* 1935; **102**: 801–13.

2.   Vineberg A, Miller G, Internal mammary coronary anastomosis in the surgical treatment

of coronary artery insufficiency, *Can Med Ass J* 1951; **64**: 204–10.

3. Favoloro RG, Saphenous vein autograft replacement of severe segmental coronary artery occlusion, *Ann Thorac Surg* 1968; **5**: 334–9.

4. European Coronary Surgery Study Group, Long-term results of prospective randomised study of coronary artery bypass surgery in stable angina pectoris, *Lancet* 1982; **ii**: 1173–80.

5. CASS Principal Investigators and their associates, Myocardial infarction and mortality in the coronary artery surgery randomized trial, *N Engl J Med* 1984; **310**: 750–8.

6. Roques F, Nashef SAM, Michel P et al, Risk factors and outcome in European cardiac surgery: analysis of the EuroSCORE multinational database of 19030 patients, *Eur J Cardiothorac Surg;* in press.

7. Parsonnet V, Dean D, Bernstein AD, A method of uniform stratification of risk for evaluating the results of surgery in acquired adult heart disease, *Circulation* 1989; **79** (suppl 1): 3–12.

8. Nashef SAM, Roques F, Michel P et al, European system for cardiac operative risk evaluation (EuroSCORE), *Eur J Cardiothorac Surg* 1999; in press.

9. Califf RM, Harrell FE Jr, Lee KL et al, Changing efficacy of coronary revascularization: implication for patient selection, *Circulation* 1988; **78** (suppl 1): 185.

10. Schofield PM, Sharples LD, Caine N et al, Transmyocardial laser revascularisation in patients with refractory angina: a randomised controlled trial, *Lancet* 1999; **353**: 519–24.

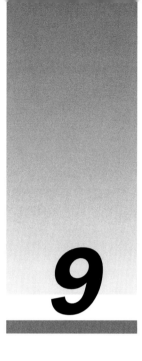

New technologies

Peter M Schofield

9

In the vast majority of patients with angina due to coronary artery disease, successful treatment can be achieved by medication, coronary angioplasty/stenting, or coronary artery bypass surgery. A few patients, however, have diffuse disease in the distal part of their coronary circulation, which is not suitable for treatment by either coronary angioplasty/stenting or coronary artery bypass grafting. These patients will often have undergone several revascularization procedures in the past. Clearly, such patients present a difficult management problem, and in recent years new laser techniques have been used for treatment. These include transmyocardial laser revascularization and percutaneous myocardial revascularization.

Transmyocardial laser revascularization (TMLR)

This technique uses laser energy to create transmural channels in the left ventricular myocardium. The concept is not a new one. Attempts were made at direct myocardial revascularization before the advent of coronary bypass surgery and coronary angioplasty.[1,2] Transmural channels were created using a variety of tubes and needles, although there was only limited clinical improvement. The concept was based on the knowledge of the myocardial sinusoids and the thebesian system—it was hoped to provide direct perfusion of the myocardium from the left ventricular cavity. In the past, direct implantation of the left internal mammary artery into the myocardium was used to encourage new vessel formation[3]—the Vineberg procedure. TMLR, at least in principle, incorporates the direct perfusion and new vessel formation of these other techniques. The exact mechanism of action of TMLR remains unknown. Direct perfusion, denervation produced by the surgical procedure and new vessel formation (angiogenesis) have all been suggested.[4] The most likely mechanism for symptomatic improvement at this stage would seem to be angiogenesis.

A left anterolateral thoracotomy is the standard approach used for TMLR, although the procedure has been performed using thoracoscopic techniques. The area(s) of ischaemia is determined preoperatively using myocardial perfusion scanning (nuclear techniques or positron emission tomography). This is exposed, having opened the pericardium and dissecting it free from the heart. Cardiopulmonary bypass is not required. The original laser used was the high-energy carbon dioxide system (The Heart Laser, PLC Medical Systems), although Holmium-YAG and Excimer lasers have also been used. The laser probe is placed onto the surface of the left ventricle and fired when the heart is maximally distended with blood and electrically quiescent, on the R wave of the electrocardiogram. The laser energy is rapidly absorbed by the blood within the left ventricle and this produces an acoustic image, analogous to steam, which is readily seen on a transoesophageal echocardiogram. The channels created by the carbon dioxide laser are approximately one millimetre in diameter and are created in a distribution of around one per square centimetre. Direct finger pressure is usually adequate to control the bleeding from the channel, although occasionally an epicardial suture is required.

Studies using the carbon dioxide laser have suggested an improvement both subjectively and objectively following TMLR. An uncontrolled, multicentre clinical trial in the USA, involving 200 patients, reported an operative mortality of 9%.[4] All of the patients had angina refractory to medical therapy, evidence of reversible myocardial ischaemia by perfusion scanning and coronary artery disease which was not suitable for conventional revascularization. There was a significant improvement in the Canadian Cardiovascular Score (CCS) for angina at 3, 6 and 12 months following the procedure. Around 75% of patients experienced a decrease of two CCS classes in their angina. There was also a significant reduction in the number of perfusion defects in the treated left ventricular wall. Prior to treatment, the number of admissions for angina was 2.5 per patient-year. This fell to 0.5 per patient-year following surgery.

The operative mortality for TMLR was 9.7 in a registry report from European and Asian centres using the CO_2 laser.[5] There was a clinically significant improvement in exercise performance, measured by treadmill exercise testing, following the procedure. Less than 50% of patients achieved an improvement of two CCS classes in their angina as compared with 75% in the USA study. A variety of complications following TMLR were reported—including perioperative bleeding and infection, left ventricular failure in the early postoperative period and both supraventricular and ventricular cardiac arrhythmias.

In recent years, TMLR has been used more widely in Europe, Asia and the USA. The potential benefits of the procedure in terms of symptomatic improvement and increased exercise capacity will need to justify the perioperative morbidity and mortality if the procedure is to become universally accepted. The results of a USA multicentre randomized controlled trial of TMLR against medical management have been submitted to the Food and Drug Administration Advisory Committee. This originally recommended non-approval for use in the USA due to the lack of a definitive explanation for the underlying mechanism, although many other well-accepted techniques in clinical practice still lack full insight into the pathophysiological mechanism. There were also concerns about the conduct of the trial in that the design allowed crossover from medical treatment to TMLR and follow-up data were incomplete. The revised submission, however, has since been approved. The UK randomized trial of TMLR against medical therapy, funded by the MRC, has now been completed. A total of 188 patients with refractory angina, evidence of reversible ischaemia on nuclear perfusion scanning and coronary artery disease not amenable to conventional revascularization were randomized. There was no crossover from medical treatment to TMLR, and follow-up was for at least 1 year. TMLR improved the CCS score for angina and increased exercise performance.[6] The perioperative mortality was 5%. There was no significant difference in myocardial perfusion between the TMLR and control groups, and no significant difference in survival at 12 months. The perioperative mortality in this trial was lower than in previously published series.[4,5] Patients with unstable angina or a left ventricular ejection fraction below 30%, however, were excluded—both of these features are known to increase the perioperative risk.

Percutaneous myocardial revascularization (PMR)

It is now possible to perform direct myocardial laser revascularization using a percutaneous approach. A Holmium-YAG laser has been developed to deliver energy directly to the endocardial surface of the left ventricle (Percutaneous Myocardial Revascularization, Cardiogenesis). This technique is much less invasive from the patient's viewpoint. There is no need for a general anaesthetic and thoracotomy, with a consequent reduction in the length of hospital stay. Following TMLR, the mean length of stay is between 10 and 12 days, whereas patients can usually be discharged from hospital 24–28 h after PMR.

Access to the left ventricle is gained via a 9 Fr sheath introduced into the femoral artery, using the Cardiogenesis PMR system. The equipment consists of a 'guiding catheter', a 'laser catheter' (which has a right-angle bend towards its tip) and a 'laser fibre' which is passed through the laser catheter (Fig. 9.1). The two views typically selected to carry out the procedure are the 40° right anterior oblique and the 50° left anterior oblique, often with up to 10° of cranial angulation. Once the views have been selected, it is essential that the patients and the X-ray table do not move. While a biplane facility is preferred, the procedure can be easily carried

out on single-plane equipment, although it may take slightly longer. The 'guiding catheter' is advanced to the left ventricular cavity, and pre-procedure left ventricular angiograms are performed in two selected views. Coronary angiograms are also carried out pre-procedure in the same projections. The coronary angiograms and the left ventricular angiograms are traced onto acetate sheets which have been fixed over the viewing screens—these than act as 'maps' during the procedure. Myocardial perfusion scanning prior to the procedure determines which area(s) is to be treated. Reversible ischaemia may be present in the anterior, inferior or lateral walls of the left ventricle or may involve the interventricular septum or left ventricular apex. All of these sites are accessible for laser treatment.

The 'laser catheter' is advanced through the 'guiding catheter' which has been positioned within the left ventricle. By manipulating the 'guiding catheter' and/or the 'laser catheter', all sites within the left ventricle can be accessed. Once the 'laser catheter' is in the appropriate position, the 'laser fibre' is advanced through the 'laser catheter' until there is a contact with the endocardial surface of the left ventricle. This can usually be felt, but can be seen radiologically as the 'laser catheter' backs away from the left ventricular wall—frequently, ventricular ectopics are produced. The right anterior oblique

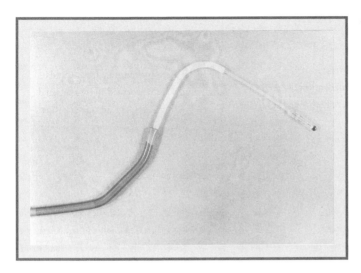

Figure 9.1
Guiding catheter/laser
catheter/laser fibre.

projection is usually preferred for demonstrating contact with the anterior and inferior walls and the left anterior oblique view for contact with the lateral and septal walls. The 'laser fibre' should be perpendicular to the left ventricular wall prior to activating the laser (Fig. 9.2). Activation of the laser usually produces 3 mm of penetration into the left ventricular myocardium. The 'laser fibre' is then advanced slightly and reactivated, which produces a channel of around 6 mm in total into the wall. The 'laser fibre' is then withdrawn into the 'laser catheter' and a new site is selected by manipulating the 'guiding catheter' and/or 'laser catheter'. In order to reduce the risk of perforation, it is important

to ensure that the area to be treated is at least 8 mm thick, using transthoracic echocardiography prior to the procedure. Once a channel has been created, the site is recorded by marking it on the acetate sheet in the two views (Fig. 9.3). Typically, channels are created at about 1 cm intervals. A total of 10–15 channels is usually created in each of the areas demonstrated to have evidence of reversible ischaemia (anterior, inferior, lateral or septal). Patients are given a bolus of heparin (usually 10 000 units) prior to the procedure. It is quite common to induce ventricular ectopics, couplets or triplets and even non-sustained ventricular tachycardia during manipulation of the 'guiding catheter'

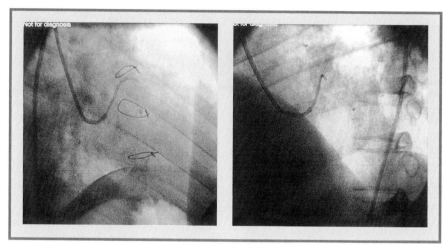

Figure 9.2
Laser fibre against the left ventricular (LV) wall. Right anterior oblique projection (left) and left anterior oblique projection (right).

and 'laser catheter'. The rhythm disturbance usually responds to repositioning of the catheters. At the moment, PMR is not used if there is evidence of left ventricular thrombus. The presence of significant aortic stenosis and severe peripheral vascular disease also precludes the use of PMR, due to problems of access to the left ventricle.

Randomized, prospective trials of PMR against medical therapy are currently in progress. These have recruited patients with refractory angina, evidence of reversible ischaemia and disease which is not suitable for conventional revascularization. The early results from non-randomized studies of PMR are encouraging. There was a significant improvement in angina class and increase in exercise test at 3 and 6 months following the procedure.[7] There are now systems other than the Cardiogenesis system in clinical trials. If PMR is shown to be effective, then it is likely to be preferred to TMLR in patients who have no other revascularization option, since it is much less invasive. TMLR, however, may still have a useful role—perhaps as an adjunct to coronary artery bypass surgery. Many patients have obstructed coronary vessels, some of

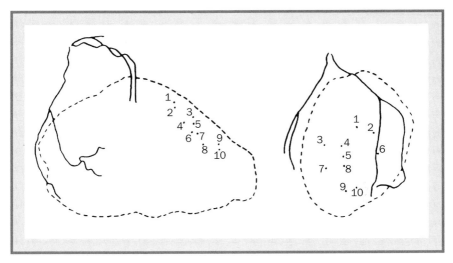

Figure 9.3
Map of channels after procedure. Right anterior oblique projection (left). Left anterior oblique projection (right).

which are suitable for bypass grafting and some of which are not. In these patients, a combined procedure of bypass surgery to some territories and TMLR to other regions may be the optimal treatment.

Other laser techniques

In interventional cardiology, the presence of a chronic totally occluded coronary artery continues to be a major problem. The procedural success rate is lower for patients with chronic total occlusions as compared with those who have stenosed, but patent, vessels. The success rate is usually in the order of 50–70%,[8,9] depending to some extent on the nature of the occlusion and its duration. Around 10% of all attempted coronary angioplasties are performed for chronic total occlusions.[10] Failure to treat such lesions may be due to the inability to cross the occlusion with a guidewire or inability to advance the balloon catheter across the occlusion once the guidewire has crossed successfully. A variety of technologies have been introduced without a major improvement in success rates. These include guidewires with olive-shaped tips, drills of various velocities, radiofrequency heat applicators and laser devices. Two laser technologies will be considered further: first, the laser guidewires, and second, the over-the-wire Excimer laser catheter.

Laser guidewires have been used for the initial passage through chronic total occlusions.[11] In some cases, an argon laser-hearted balltip (hot tip) guidewire has been successful when conventional systems have failed. Vessel perforation is a possible complication of the technique, and this technology is now rarely used. The results of the bare argon laser instrument (Lastac) are comparable to those using less costly mechanical methods.[12] There is a beneficial mechanical component with these catheters, which have features that may be useful when treating chronic total occlusions—stiffness and bluntness. There is a lack of randomized clinical trials against conventional technologies, and this equipment now has very limited application.

The use of the Excimer laser catheter requires the passage of a guidewire through the chronic total occlusion, which, clearly, is not always possible. Once the guidewire has been advanced through the occlusion to the distal vessel, the Excimer laser catheter can be used to ablate tissue. The system can be used with over-the-wire multifibre catheters of different diameters. Generally, the larger the diameter

of the vessel being treated, the larger the diameter of the laser catheter utilized. Having crossed the total occlusion with a guidewire, the Excimer laser catheter is advanced to the lesion. During laser ablation, the catheter is advanced slowly—at about 1 mm/s. The initial laser procedure may produce an acceptable angiographic result, or it may be necessary to sequentially increase the catheter size, or it may be necessary to use conventional angioplasty technology (i.e. balloon catheters or stents) to produce an optimal result.

Results from the Excimer Laser Coronary Angioplasty Registry indicated that once a guidewire crossed the total occlusion, the overall success rate of the procedure was 83%.[13] In 74% of patients, adjunctive balloon angioplasty was used after laser treatment. The results indicate that Excimer laser angioplasty may be useful for treating chronic total occlusions that can be crossed with a guidewire but not with a balloon catheter, particularly if the occlusion is extremely long. An alternative strategy when treating occlusions which can be crossed with a guidewire but not the balloon catheter is to use the Rotablator system—this is discussed below.

Conventional balloon angioplasty improves luminal dimensions by producing fracture of the atheromatous plaque and stretching the plaque-free wall. The aim of laser balloon angioplasty is to create a large, smooth vascular lumen by thermal welding. In theory, this could potentially reduce the occurrence of dissection flaps, eliminate vascular recoil, reduce coronary vasospasm and inhibit platelet activation and smooth muscle cell proliferation.[14] Laser balloon angioplasty permits the application of heat (generated by the laser source) and pressure (by balloon inflations) to thermally weld tissue during coronary angioplasty. The system uses a Nd:YAG laser and a modified coronary angioplasty catheter with a PET balloon. The technique is very similar to conventional balloon angioplasty. Once in the appropriate position, the balloon is inflated to low pressure (usually about 4 atmospheres) and the laser dose is delivered over about 20 s. This results in adventitial temperatures of between 90°C and 110°C. The balloon inflation is then continued for a further 40 s while the temperature of the arterial wall returns to normal.

Laser balloon angioplasty has been shown to be effective in the management of acute failure of balloon coronary angioplasty, due either to immediate vessel recoil or severe dissection with impaired flow ('impending closure'). Despite a high early success rate, however, the late angiographic restenosis rate of laser balloon angioplasty is similar to that of conventional balloon angioplasty.[14] With the introduction of coronary stents, the

potential role for laser balloon angioplasty seems to have been taken over. Coronary stents can be used to treat the acute problems of vessel recoil and severe dissection. In addition, coronary stents are associated with a lower late angiographic restenosis rate. Therefore, laser balloon angioplasty now has very limited application.

Directional atherectomy

This technique involves the removal of tissue from the diseased coronary artery. It was hoped that by debulking the lesion and removing atheroma, the incidence of restenosis would be reduced. The original directional atherectomy catheters were quite large and stiff. They required the use of an 8 Fr or 9 Fr guiding catheter and could not usually be advanced to the more distal parts of the coronary circulation. The atherectomy catheter is advanced to the lesion over a guidewire and has a balloon attached to the housing of the cutter (Fig. 9.4). Inflation of the balloon pushes the device against the wall of the diseased vessel, and the atheromatous tissue 'falls' into the window in the housing. The cutter is then activated and advanced within the housing, 'slicing off' the atherematous tissue, which is then stored in the 'nosecone' of the device. Several cuts can be made around the circumference of the vessel by rotating the device. The device can be used in large-calibre vessels which are

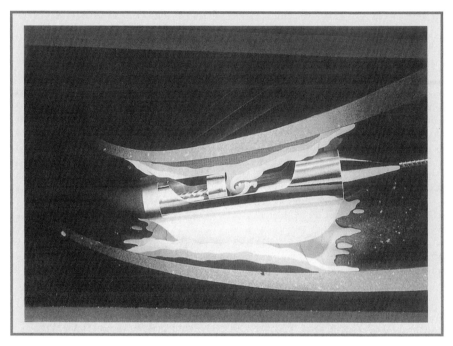

Figure 9.4
Atherectomy device.

reasonably straight—particularly if the atheroma is eccentric.

The use of directional atherectomy has declined since randomized studies reported that there was no reduction in angiographic restenosis by directional atherectomy as compared with balloon angioplasty.[15] There were also some concerns in respect of late complications following atherectomy—in particular coronary aneurysm formation. The situation has been re-evaluated using small devices,[16] but as yet no clear advantage of atherectomy over angioplasty/stenting has been demonstrated. Atherectomy has been a valuable research tool, allowing removal of tissue from lesions for further study. These lesions may be 'de novo' atheromatous lesions, restenotic lesions following balloon angioplasty and 'in-stent' restenotic lesions following coronary stenting.

Rotablator

The Rotablator device enables high-speed rotational atherectomy. The device is advanced over a guidewire and has an olive tip which is coated with diamond chips. The olive tip is available in a range of diameters, the size being determined by the size of the vessel to be treated. An external motor rotates the device at speeds of around 180 000 rev/min. Not surprisingly, use of the device may be associated with severe coronary spasm, particularly in the distal coronary artery beyond the lesion. Patients are therefore given intracoronary nitrate and/or verapamil during the procedure to reduce the problem of spasm.

The Rotablator device has been used in a variety of situations. It may be useful when treating lesions which can be crossed with a guidewire, but not the balloon catheter, or when the balloon catheter 'fails to dilate' the diseased segment despite the use of high inflation pressures. By using catheters of progressively increasing burr-size, an acceptable angiographic result can be achieved using the Rotablator alone. Usually, however, balloon angioplasty/stenting is required following rotablation in order to achieve a good angiographic result. The device may be useful for treating heavily calcified lesions, since it may fracture the calcium and reduce the risk of dissection with subsequent balloon

dilatation. It may also be useful when treating lesions at the ostium of a coronary artery or with diffusely diseased vessels.[17] More recently, the device has been used to treat restenosis within coronary stents. This is a difficult disease process to treat, and randomized prospective trials are in progress. Although the Rotablator device at the moment has only a fairly limited application, it will probably be used more widely than the directional atherectomy catheter. If the device is shown to offer advantages in the treatment of 'in-stent' restenosis, then its use will increase substantially.

Intravascular ultrasound

This form of imaging has great potential to assist during angioplasty and aid in the assessment of coronary artery disease. Whereas coronary angiography studies the lumen of the vessel, intravascular ultrasound provides information on the wall of the vessel. There are two methods of generating the images: first, a mechanical approach using a rotating mirror, and second, a phased array system. The ultrasound catheter is passed down the coronary artery over a routine angioplasty guidewire. Many of the intravascular ultrasound systems can be used in conjunction with a 'pull-back' device. This withdraws the catheter at a slow constant speed which results in a better recording of the images which are generated (Fig. 9.5).

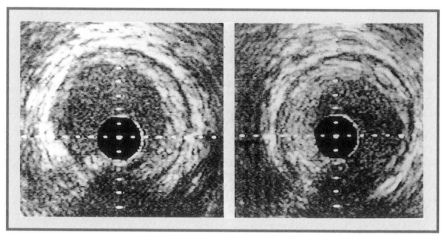

Figure 9.5
IVUS image showing marked intimal hyperplasia in a patient following cardiac transplantation.

Intravascular ultrasound may be useful to confirm full expansion of a coronary artery stent, and to assess in-stent restenosis, since it may demonstrate incomplete stent expansion or intimal hyperplasia. It is useful for accurately measuring the size of the vessel lumen. Often, the size of the vessel measured by intravascular ultrasound is greater than the calibre demonstrated by angiography: this may be helpful when treating restenotic lesions. Intravascular ultrasound is more sensitive than angiography for the demonstration of vascular calcification and may be useful for the assessment of coronary artery lesions involving the bifurcation of vessels.

It has been suggested that intravascular ultrasound will help in deciding on the strategy to be used during interventional procedures. For example, the presence of extensive vascular calcification may indicate the need for the initial use of the Rotablator device. In most units, however, the technology is not widely used. It has a role to play in terms of research projects involving the assessment of coronary artery disease. With the introduction of newer, more conformable coronary stents, the requirement for the routine use of intravascular ultrasound to confirm adequate deployment has decreased markedly.

References

1. Sen PK, Udwadia TE, Kinare SG et al, Transmyocardial acupuncture: a new approach to myocardial revascularisation, *J Thorac Cardiovasc Surg* 1965; **50**: 181–9.

2. Khazei AH, Kime WP, Papadopoulos C et al, Myocardial canalization: a new method of myocardial revascularisation, *Ann Thorac Surg* 1968; **6**: 163–71.

3. Vineberg A, Clinical and experimental studies in the treatment of coronary artery insufficiency by internal mammary artery implant, *J Int Coll Surg* 1954; **22**: 503–18.

4. Horvath KA, Cohn LH, Cooley DA, Transmyocardial laser revascularisation: results of a multicentre trial with transmyocardial laser revascularisation used as sole therapy for end-stage coronary artery disease, *J Thorac Cardiovasc Surg* 1997; **113**: 645–54.

5. Burns SM, Sharpleas LD, Tait S et al, The transmyocardial laser revascularisation international registry report, *Eur Heart J* 1999; **20**: 31–7.

6. Schofield PM, Sharples LO, Caine N et al. The UK randomized controlled trial of transmyocardial revascularization in patients with refractory angina. *Lancet* 1999; **353**: 519–24.

7. Lauer B, Junghans U, Stahl F, Kluge R, Oesterle S, Sculer G, Catheter-based percutaneous myocardial laser revascularisation in patients with end-stage coronary artery disease. *Eur Heart J* 1998; **589** (abstract).

8. Hamm CW, Kupper W, Kuck K, Hofmann D, Bleifeld W, Recanalisation of chronic totally occluded coronary arteries by new angioplasty systems, *Am J Cardiol* 1990; **66**: 1459–63.

9. Bell MR, Berger PB, Bresnahan JF, Reeder GS, Bailey KR, Holmes DR, Initial and long-term outcome of 354 patients after coronary balloon angioplasty of total coronary artery occlusions, *Circulation* 1992; **85**: 1003–11.

10. Detre K, Hobkov R, Kelsey S et al, Percutaneous transluminal coronary angioplasty in 1985–88 and 1977–81. The National Heart, Lung and Blood Institute Registry, *N Engl J Med* 1988; **318**: 265–70.

11. Bowes RJ, Oakley GD, Fleming JS et al, Early clinical experience with a hot tip laser wire in patients with chronic coronary artery occlusion, *J Invas Cardiol* 1990; **2**: 241–5.

12. Mast EG, Plokker HW, Ernst JM et al, Percutaneous recanalisation of chronic total occlusions: experience with the direct Argon laser assisted angioplasty system (LASTAC), *Herz* 1990; **15**: 241–4.

13. Holmes DR, Forrester JS, Litvack F et al, Chronic total obstruction and short-term outcome: the Excimer laser coronary angioplasty registry experience, *Mayo Clin Proc* 1993; **68**: 5–10.

14. Safian RD, Reis GJ, Pomerantz RM, Laser balloon angioplasty: potential clinical applications, *Herz* 1990; **15**: 299–306.

15. Topol EJ, Leya F, Pinkerton CA et al, A comparison of directional atherectomy with coronary angioplasty in patients with coronary artery disease. The CAVEAT trial, *N Engl J Med* 1993; **329**: 221–7.

16. Dussaillant GR, Mintz GS, Popma JJ et al, Intravascular ultrasound, directional atherectomy and the optimal atherectomy restenosis study (OARS), *Coronary Artery Dis* 1996; **7**: 294–8.

17. MacIsaac AI, Bass TA, Buchbinder M et al, High speed rotational atherectomy: outcome in calcified and non-calcified coronary artery lesions, *J Am Coll Cardiol* 1995; **30**: 731–6.

Index